The Plot Against the *NHS*

Colin Leys &
Stewart Player

The Plot
Against
the *NHS*

MERLIN PRESS

© Colin Leys and Stewart Player, 2011

Cartoon pp. vi and 154
© Julian Tudor Hart

First published in 2011 by
The Merlin Press Ltd.
6 Crane Street Chambers
Crane Street
Pontypool
NP4 6ND
Wales

www.merlinpress.co.uk

ISBN. 978-0-85036-679-2

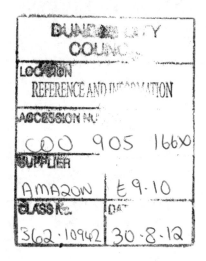
British Library Cataloguing in Publication Data
is available from the British Library

Printed in UK by Imprint Digital, Exeter

Contents

List of acronyms

A and E   Accident and Emergency
APMS   Alternative Provider Medical Services
BMA   British Medical Association
BMJ   British Medical Journal
CBI   Confederation of British Industry
CEO   Chief Executive Officer
CfH   Connecting for Health
CHC   Community Health Council
GP   General Practitioner
HMO   Health Maintenance Organization
ISTC   Independent Sector Treatment Centre
IT   Information Technology
LIFT   Local Investment Finance Trust
LINk   Local Involvement Network
PCT   Primary Care Trust
PFI   Private Finance Initiative
QOF   Quality Outcomes Framework
TUC   Trade Union Congress

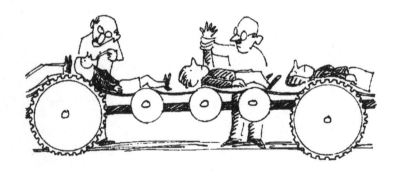

Foreword

Dr Jacky Davis, MBBS, FRCR

'Since 2000 governments have pursued a policy for the NHS that the electorate hasn't voted for and doesn't want'. This timely book seeks to explain how and why this has happened, how politicians and private interests have worked patiently together behind closed doors to try to transform the NHS from an integrated public service into a mere 'kitemark' attached to a system of competing private providers.

The NHS – one of the most cost effective and equitable health services in the world – now stands on the brink of extinction, and many will be waking up and wondering how we arrived at this point without an outcry from the public and the media. This book takes the apparently disparate pieces of the jigsaw puzzle and fits them together to give us the bigger picture. And the picture that emerges is of a popular and effective public service betrayed by corporate greed and political dishonesty.

The book looks at how this subterfuge was possible. Politicians have increasingly made cause with the private sector, opening the door to commercial interests through step by step reforms, each of which has concealed its true purpose in language with which we have become only too familiar. We have been lulled by talk of patient choice, modernisation, world class commissioning, contestability and plurality of providers. Politicians have hardly ever used the word 'market', and the intention to privatize has always been denied.

The authors take us through the history of the NHS 'reforms', whereby the mechanisms of the market –

foundation trusts, payment by results, commissioning Primary Care Trusts – were put in place behind a smokescreen of spin, bogus public consultations, distortion of the truth and outright lies. The penetration of the Department of Health by the private health lobby is exposed, as well as the 'revolving door' between government and the corporate sector. Importantly, the book describes what the brave new world of a healthcare market will look like to patients in the NHS of tomorrow.

This book should be read by anyone with an interest in the NHS – by the taxpayers who fund it, by those who work in it and by those who rely on it. It gives us a clear picture of where the NHS now stands and how it got here. This compelling analysis means that we can be under no illusion about the intentions of politicians and the medical industrial complex. It is up to us now to do something about it.

Preface

This book should have been written at least six months sooner, but we believed David Cameron when he promised during the 2010 election that if the Conservatives were elected there would be 'no top-down reorganization of the NHS'. We were naive. Now that Andrew Lansley's bill is before parliament, people have begun to see what is in store.

We have tried to show what has been happening, and why it is important. What is intended is the end of the NHS as a universal public service and its replacement by a healthcare market, driven by the search for profits. No one can say that isn't important. The NHS has been a fundamental component of social solidarity and equal citizenship for over sixty years. If it goes we will eventually find ourselves living in a very different kind of society.

So this book has been written for everyone who feels the need for a health service that is truly comprehensive and free; and for one they can trust, as opposed to having to confront a marketplace of health 'products' and providers and never knowing if what is being offered is really in their interest, or the interest of shareholders. It is especially written for everyone who feels *entitled* to the NHS, and is not willing to see it abolished by politicians who have no mandate to do any such thing.

Thanks are due to the NHS Consultants' Association for permission to use data from Stewart Player's 2010 report, 'Reshaping the NHS and its Implications for Consultants', and to the Andrew Wainwright Reform Trust and the Lipman-Miliband Trust for generous financial support. Particular thanks are due to Stuart Jeffery and Barbara Harriss-White for important comments and criticisms, and to Lynn Spink for good advice and expert editing of the whole text. We are also indebted to Tamasin Cave at Spinwatch, Matthew Dunnigan and Jonathon Tomlinson for invaluable contributions on particular issues, and to Julian Tudor Hart for insisting on the importance of what has been happening in Scotland, Wales and Northern Ireland, for helping us with information on Wales, and for allowing us to use his iconic illustration of the concept of efficiency that underlies the market model. Above all we are indebted to Sally Ruane and David Rowland, who generously put their expertise at our disposal with penetrating and often challenging comments on every chapter. We alone, however, are responsible for all remaining errors, and for all the opinions we express. Thanks finally also to Tony Zurbrugg and Adrian Howe at the Merlin Press for their steady support and for bringing the book out in a reader-friendly format and at record speed.

When we think of the next generation, to whom we should be leaving an NHS as excellent and free as it has been for us, we think especially of Merlie, Patrick, Trixie, Cora, Daisy and Isabel, and dedicate the book to them.

1

The Plot

Plot: *a secret plan, esp. to achieve an unlawful end; a conspiracy;* Conspiracy: *combination of people for an unlawful or reprehensible purpose.*

(Oxford English Dictionary)

In July 2000 the Independent Healthcare Association, representing Britain's still very modest – by international standards – private healthcare industry, was in the middle of negotiating a 'concordat' with Tony Blair's second Secretary of State for Health, Alan Milburn. The Association's leading negotiator, Tim Evans, was very clear on the ultimate aim of the concordat. He looked forward, he said, 'to a time when the NHS would simply be a kitemark attached to the institutions and activities of a system of purely private providers'.[1]

At the time this sounded like the kind of fantasy you might expect from a policy adviser to the far-right Adam Smith Institute, which Evans also was. The NHS was still a taken-for-granted fixture of British life and values. But less than three months later a concordat was reached to make private companies permanent providers of treatment to NHS patients. By 2009, 149 private hospitals, 'treatment centres' and clinics were treating NHS patients 'on the NHS', and using the NHS logo.

By 2014, if Cameron's and Lansley's Health and Social Care Bill becomes law, the remaining NHS hospital trusts, mental health trusts, ambulance trusts and the rest will all have been converted into independent businesses, increasingly indistinguishable from private companies. They will be competing in a market, in which the penalty for financial failure will be either closing, or being taken over by a private company.[2] A growing number of nominally NHS hospitals are also expected to be under private sector management. Indeed under the new Bill there is nothing to stop all NHS services being taken over by private providers.

Of course the fact that the privatizers' dream is so close to being realized, and so astonishingly soon, isn't evidence of a plot or conspiracy. Breaking up the NHS and replacing it with a healthcare market was not an illegal aim, or even reprehensible, at least in the eyes of those involved. In a democracy everyone is free to pursue their own interests and preferences.

Yet it was a plot. What made it a plot was its covert nature. Neither parliament nor the public have ever been told honestly what was intended. Misrepresentation, obfuscation and deception have been involved at every stage.

Opinion polls show that at any time since 2000, if the public had been asked whether they wanted to see the NHS broken up and replaced with a healthcare market on American lines, to be run for profit by a variety of multinational health companies, private equity funds and local businessmen, they would have overwhelmingly rejected it.[3] If the idea had been openly put before parliament only a handful of Conservative MPs in very safe seats could have risked supporting it. Whatever its faults, the NHS remains the most popular institution in the country. So if the project was to succeed it was essential to minimize public attention to what was really intended – and when attention could not be avoided, to obscure it.

The year 2000 presented the marketizers with an unprecedented opportunity. By promising a massive one-third real-terms increase in NHS funding, to be achieved over the next five years, bringing it up to the EU average, Tony Blair made available money that could spent on creating a market without seeming to be at the expense of urgently-needed services.

The increase was intended to remove the valid complaint by NHS staff and others that the service's fundamental problem was chronic underfunding.

Among other things NHS staff received substantial pay rises – in the case of most GPs, a dramatic rise. In return Blair asked the leaders of the NHS to sign up to a new 'NHS Plan', which called for radical improvements in the way services should be run, patients treated, complaints handled, and so on.[4] A long list of senior doctors, nurses, managers and others were happy to sign. Most of the aims made sense, and with new resources they thought they could be achieved.

The NHS Plan was packaged as being about 'modernizing' the NHS, making it more efficient and more responsive to patients' needs. It said nothing about a healthcare market. It did say that the time had now come 'to engage more constructively with the private sector' and end the 'standoff' which had existed between it and the NHS for decades. It said that 'ideological boundaries or institutional barriers should not stand in the way of better care for NHS patients' and the NHS should 'harness the capacity of private and voluntary (meaning private non-profit) providers to treat more NHS patients'. And a section towards the end announced the new concordat, which Milburn was in the process of finalizing.

The concordat suggested that the private sector might provide the NHS with more services, such as pathology, imaging and dialysis, but as regards treating patients the only suggestion was that more regular use might be made of private hospitals to take advantage of their spare capacity. Nowhere did the NHS Plan even hint at the possibility of making the NHS into a mere kitemark applied to a system of for-profit companies.

Four years later the government published an NHS Improvement Plan which focused on 'patient choice' and said that by 2008 there would be a 'growing range of independent sector providers' for NHS patients, providing up to 15 per cent of all 'elective', non-emergency procedures. But there was still no suggestion that this was meant to be a stage in the conversion of the NHS into a full healthcare market.[5]

Yet behind the scenes key policy-makers were working precisely towards that end, creating one opening for the private sector after another – in ways that had indeed been sketched in the NHS Plan, though without spelling out their real implications. By 2004, in fact, all the main elements of a market were in place – Primary Care Trusts acting as commissioners, foundation trusts competing with a gradually widening range of private providers, treatments priced and paid for patient by patient, and the beginnings of an IT-based system of patient choice.

Glimpses of what was intended did surface occasionally. John Reid, when he was Secretary of State for Health, caused a brief commotion when he said NHS hospitals that failed to attract patients would close;[6] and his successor Patricia Hewitt did the same when she said that there was no upper limit to the percentage of NHS work that could be given to the private sector.[7]

But these public admissions, prompted by the need to keep the private sector sweet in face of what it saw as a far too sluggish rate of progress towards a market, were soon forgotten. As a result very few people understood what was really intended by the strategists inside the Department of Health. When Andrew Lansley's White Paper of July 2010 revealed what was really in store many MPs, and even many doctors, struggled to comprehend it.

So in spite of its great popularity Britain's most famous postwar social achievement was unravelled through a series of step-by-step 'reforms', each creating the basis for the next one, and always presented as mere improvements to the NHS as a public service. They were billed as measures to reduce waiting times, to offer more 'choice', to achieve 'world class' standards, to make the NHS more 'patient-centred' – anything but the real underlying aim of the key strategists involved, to turn health care back into a commodity and a source of profit.

Each of the so-called reforms involved persistent, behind-the-scenes lobbying and fixing by a network of insiders – inside the Department of Health, above all, but also by a wider network, closely linked to the Department: corporate executives, management consultants, ministers' 'special advisers', academics with free market sympathies and a taste for power, doctors with entrepreneurial ambitions – and the House of Commons Health Committee, packed with just enough compliant back-benchers and deliberately insulated from advice from expert critics of the market agenda. Not to mention a large and growing corporate lobby.

Each 'reform' needed its own quantum of dissimulation and occasionally downright lies. The culture of the Department of Health was radically transformed. In place of old-fashioned ideas of accountability and fidelity to facts the priority shifted to misrepresentation and spin. This was accelerated by the fact that from the late 1990s onwards more and more private sector personnel were active inside the Department, often in leading roles.

Many were initially involved as consultants on PFI (Private Finance Initiative) hospital contracts, which the government made clear was the only way a hospital could be rebuilt or replaced. By 2010 a total of 103 PFI hospital schemes, originally valued at £11.3 billion, but expected to cost £65 billion over their lifetimes, had been completed or were in progress.[8] To get a PFI contract the PFI way of financing had to look better 'value for money' than using publicly borrowed finance, and this led to systematic manipulation of the figures. Even the Deputy Controller and Auditor-General admitted that this involved 'pseudo-scientific mumbo-jumbo' in which 'if the answer comes out wrong you don't get your project. So the answer doesn't come out wrong very often.'[9] Civil servants had to unlearn some long-established principles of objectivity and honesty in order to sign off on PFI projects.

And after the year 2000 large numbers of private sector staff were directly employed by the Department. Departmental documents increasingly looked and read like business promotional material. Divining their real meaning called for the skills of a cold war-era Kremlin-watcher.

What lay behind the marketization drive? The interests of the corporate health industry – global as much as British – were obvious. The huge NHS budget, with its assured flow of tax revenues, was of intense interest not only to healthcare multinationals such as the American Health Maintenance Organization (HMO) UnitedHealth and the South African hospital chain Netcare, but also to companies such as Atos

Origin, a French software multi-national, and to various private equity companies equally lacking in any healthcare background – as well as to dozens of smaller British firms, all keen to get in on the act. The interest was not all on one side. Several ministers and numerous civil servants left to take highly-paid jobs in the private healthcare sector. But not all ministers and civil servants saw a financial advantage for themselves. What motivated the rest to join in?

There is no doubt that in 2000 the NHS was in need of modernization, and no one should underestimate the scale of the task, even when very substantial additional funding was made available. The NHS is a huge and complex system, consisting of 1.3 million people working in hundreds of national, regional and local organizations, with diverse job categories and subcultures and interrelationships. Millions of people depend on it to help them deal with some of the most troubling and even life-threatening problems they confront. It can't be lightly tampered with and so it poses a huge challenge to anyone trying to change it.

One can understand how politicians and officials, impatient with the pace of wished-for improvements, could be tempted by the idea that the pressure of competition could achieve what they found so difficult to achieve with the financial and administrative levers at their disposal. The message they constantly heard from businessmen was that they could accomplish in a week, with one hand tied behind their backs, what NHS managers seemed unable to do in a year, or even five.

Many strategists within the Department of Health were attracted by the notion that they could import elements of market-based healthcare systems elsewhere which looked to them more efficient, and use them to 'gee up' the surrounding structures of the NHS, without going all the way to a full-scale market. Such policy-makers can be thought of as 'marketizers', in the sense that they wanted the NHS to operate more like a market, while remaining publicly funded and managed. Others can be better thought of as 'privatizers' like Tim Evans, who thought that only private companies competing in a full healthcare market would achieve the desired efficiencies.

Unfortunately the marketizers continued to advocate market models of care even when experiments showed that market-based imports were not efficient at all – as with UnitedHealth's 'Evercare' programme, for example. Evercare, which the huge American HMO UnitedHealth was paid a large sum to test in four regions of England, was supposed to reduce emergency hospital admissions for elderly patients by 50 per cent. But when it was evaluated it turned out to be unlikely to cut admissions by more than one per cent.[10] The marketizers had evidently not reckoned with the fact that England's system of primary care was already accomplishing what Evercare does in the US, where there is no free primary care. The main lesson the Department of Health seemed to draw from this experience was not to evaluate such experiments.

Besides being ready to ignore evidence, many of the marketizers in the Department, and their academic and think-tank advisers, also imagined that the state would always set limits on the role of market forces. They thought market forces would always operate 'within a planned and managed system', as Labour's shadow health secretary, John Healey, put it in the Commons in February 2011.[11] They assumed that 'the power of the markets' could be 'harnessed' to drive needed improvements in the NHS, without market forces becoming too strong to be kept within a planned and managed system.

Perhaps they also imagined that the Conservatives would never return to power and complete the conversion of marketization into privatization.

Probably few of the strategists under Milburn and his New Labour successors were committed privatizers from the start, although some undoubtedly were. But as the decade progressed the distinction became less and less meaningful. Policy-makers abandoned their critical role and talked in increasingly vague terms about 'the direction of travel', avoiding the need to say what the destination was. As more and more NHS activities were handed over to private enterprise the companies involved were described as part of 'the NHS family'. Among policy-makers the notion that the NHS might end up as no more than a kitemark gradually ceased to be unthinkable.

By 2010 marketization clearly entailed not just the possibility but the longer-run probability of privatization. Yet the fact remains that all the evidence shows that privatization makes health care more costly – and worse. The evidence from the US confirms what economic theory says, that markets will not produce good health care for all, as the NHS is pledged to do.

A Treasury document published in 2003 clearly outlined the reasons why this is so: price signals don't work in relation to health care; the consumer lacks the necessary knowledge, creating a risk of overtreatment; there is a potential abuse of monopoly power; it is hard to write and enforce contracts for medical treatment; and 'it is difficult to let failing hospitals go bust – individuals are entitled to expect continuous, high-quality health care wherever they are'.[12]

Why was all this ignored? If the strategists in the Department of Health thought they had contrary evidence or superior theory they should have come out openly and said so. But they were never called on to defend their ideas, precisely because they proceeded so covertly.

A 2010 survey of 20,000 patients in eleven industrialised countries for the US Commonwealth Fund found that the NHS was almost the least costly healthcare system of them all, and at the same time gave one of the best levels of access to care. Other countries not only spent more per head but also charged patients directly, reducing equality of access. Only Switzerland reported faster access to care, but Switzerland also spent some 35 per cent more per head than the UK. Only New Zealand spent less per head, but one in seven New Zealanders said they skipped hospital visits because of cost. In the US, which spent almost twice as much per head as the UK, one in three people avoided seeking care because of cost.[13] To ignore all this evidence and embrace the idea of replacing one of the most cost-efficient health systems in the world, as well as one of the fairest, with one modelled on the most expensive and unequal system (the American), sets a new standard for ideologically-driven (and interest-driven) policy-making.

But the NHS has not only worked well, providing high-quality, equal care for everyone, free of charge, at low cost: it is also the historic achievement of millions of people – those who fought to establish it, those who have spent their lives working for it, and everyone who has paid their taxes to build it up over the more than sixty years since it was created. Its founding principles of comprehensiveness and equal access for all have been core values of modern British society. Working to marketize it, and finally privatizing it, without any democratic mandate – without even explaining that aim to parliament or the public, is as close as it gets to being not just unscrupulous, but actually unconstitutional. The question is whether the English people – Scotland, Wales and Northern Ireland having escaped the plotters' reach – will accept having this precious part of our heritage filched from under our noses.

2

Fragmenting the NHS and creating a market

The Independent Healthcare Association was dissolved in 2004. Tim Evans had already moved on to pursue a career as a free-market publicist at the Cobden Centre and the Adam Smith Institute.[1] Once the concordat with the government had been secured the big healthcare companies such as Norwich Union and the General Healthcare Group had no further interest in teaming up with the host of little ones that made up most of the Association's membership. They had their eyes on bigger things.

From their point of view the concordat was only a prelude to opening up the NHS to private providers on a significant scale – a view shared by the chief marketizers in the government, especially Tony Blair and his senior health adviser, Simon Stevens; Alan Milburn and his main adviser, Paul Corrigan; and Dr Penny Dash, Head of Strategy and Planning in the Department of Health.

Three crucial steps needed to be taken next. First, openings had to be created for private companies to provide health care – clinical treatments – for NHS patients on the regular basis alluded to in the concordat.

Second, NHS organizations had to be reorganized into

competitive businesses. In the 1990s under John Major most NHS bodies had been made into trusts, run by boards of governors and chief executives, which 'sold' their services to 'purchasers' in a different part of the NHS. But this so-called internal market was not a real market. The contracts made between NHS hospital trusts and local Primary Care Trusts (the so-called purchasers, or commissioners) were not legally binding. There were no major penalties for hospital trusts that failed to deliver all the treatments they had contracted to provide, or underestimated what it would cost to deliver them. If they ran into debt the management would be criticized, or might even be replaced, but money would be found to keep the trust going.

So the financial discipline that comes with the fear of going bust was missing: the needs of patients could still be seen as more important than the bottom line. If NHS hospitals and other NHS organizations, from mental health trusts to ambulance services, were to be ready to compete in a real market (and if private health companies were to be willing to compete with them), this had to change.

Third, a growing percentage of the NHS workforce had to be made ready to transfer – voluntarily or otherwise – to private sector employment. All three steps were implicit in the NHS Plan. All of them were put in hand by Alan Milburn, who had made the concordat with the private sector and presided over the Plan's drafting.

Creating entry-points for the private sector: Ken Anderson and the Commercial Directorate

Paradoxically, the immediate problem confronting the marketizers was that although the concordat said private companies could now have long-term contracts with the NHS, in practice none of them could compete with NHS hospitals at NHS prices. The NHS was not perfect (can anyone name a big organization that is?) but it provided a standard of health care for everyone that was among the best in the world, and it was also one of the least costly.

British private hospitals, by contrast, were very expensive. They depended wholly on the part-time work of NHS consultants, who demanded extremely high fees;[2] and their clientele of privately-insured patients was limited, so there were few economies of scale. No private hospital in England offered a full range of services from accident and emergency to intensive care and all major specialties. Most of their business was routine elective surgery.

To call into existence a new kind of private healthcare company capable of competing with NHS hospitals and clinics the Department of Health decided to 'unbundle' some of the most potentially lucrative, standardized, high-volume and low-risk treatments provided in NHS hospitals, and offer private companies extremely favourable terms to provide them. Cataract surgery and hip and knee replacements were the obvious treatments to start with.

The NHS had already begun to establish what the Americans rather alarmingly called 'focused factories', i.e. clinics for surgery of this kind that were separated from other surgical work, with dedicated surgical teams. In 2002 sixteen were in operation. But waiting times were still long, so inviting private providers to do the same could be represented as being designed primarily to help by bringing in 'additional capacity' from the private sector.

The man appointed to make this happen was Ken Anderson, a Texan business executive with a background in the private health sector, and most recently in the UK facilities management company, AMEY. In 2003 he was made Director-General of a new Commercial Directorate inside the Department of Health, with the brief of 'introducing independent sector providers to the NHS'. By 2006 the Directorate was an organization of 190 people, no less than 182 of whom were 'interims' – i.e. people recruited on short-term contracts from the private sector (at a daily cost to the NHS of £1,000-2,000 each).[3]

By mid-2009 the Independent Sector Treatment Centre (ISTC) programme had got some 30 privately-owned surgical centres up and running throughout England. The Department of Health's formula was that they were part of 'the NHS family'. They were allowed to use the NHS logo (kitemark), so most patients were (and still are) not aware that they are private companies.

Anderson told MPs on the House of Commons Health Committee that 'local health economies' had been involved in planning the new centres, but neither hospital doctors nor GPs in the chosen areas were seriously consulted.[4] And there was a further difficulty. Although Anderson's Commercial Directorate had planned the centres, the contracts had to be with the local Primary Care Trusts, and some members of their boards of management objected. They realized that the new centres would take income away from the local NHS providers and put other local services in jeopardy, and so they opposed signing the contracts.

But the reality was that PCTs were instruments of the Secretary of State for Health, with a veneer of local representation. This became clear when Milburn's successor, John Reid, did the necessary arm-twisting. He threatened to dismiss the chairs of dissident PCTs and surcharge their board members.[5] The board of South-West Oxfordshire PCT, which had refused to sign a contract for cataract removals that seemed bound to lead to the closure of a highly-regarded local NHS eye unit, was told that 'John Reid wanted a reversal of the decision on his desk by 12 o'clock on the Monday'. A survey of over a hundred NHS chief executives found that this was not an isolated case: the ISTC programme was 'forced through by bullying'.[6]

And so the first privately-owned, for-profit providers of NHS-funded health care started work, creating bridgeheads for the private sector that could later be steadily widened. While the scale of the work that would be undertaken by ISTCs was very small – as late as 2008 it barely exceeded two per cent of the 8.6 million elective procedures performed on NHS patients – it was remarkably costly.[7]

The main justification for the programme was that securing additional capacity from private companies would help reduce waiting lists. Providing additional capacity, however, was supposed to mean just that: the work could not be done by NHS staff. However this restriction was steadily diluted. By August 2007 ISTCs were free to use NHS staff in most clinical specialties, and were doing so. The programme's dependence on NHS staff made it clear that privatization on a larger scale would mean the permanent transfer of NHS staff to private employers.

The ISTC programme also took funding away from the NHS. In order to make it attractive to the private sector, the companies concerned were paid for the number of treatments contracted for, whether or not they were actually carried out, and at a significantly higher price than NHS providers received. In effect it was financially risk-free. Clinical risk – the risk of law-suits for medical malpractice if things went wrong – was also covered by the NHS. The money involved – £5.6 billion over 5 years – involved a significant subtraction from the NHS's resources. Its main contribution was to fatten the balance sheets of Netcare, Capio, Clinicenta and the other new private providers, feather-bedding their initial entry into the new NHS-funded healthcare market.

It was true that ISTCs offered some patients quicker access to treatment, and in new and clean environments. But NHS treatment centres were already doing this, and at considerably lower cost, in spite of having to operate on more difficult cases than the ISTCs were willing to accept. The money spent on ISTCs could have been given to local NHS providers to tackle the backlog of elective procedures far more cheaply.

Besides the alleged aim of reducing waiting lists Anderson and Ricketts admitted to MPs in the Commons Health Committee that a second objective was to offer patients 'choice', and to use competition to 'drive up standards' in the NHS. Most patients don't want a choice of providers, if that means for-profit providers.[8] But you can't have a market without people choosing between different suppliers, so patients had to be induced to choose, and GPs had to be induced to refer patients to private providers. Some GPs were even paid a bonus for every patient they referred to the local ISTC rather than the local NHS hospital.[9]

While listening politely to tall stories about 'additional capacity' told them by Anderson and Ricketts, members of the Commons Health Committee were subjected to extraordinary teasing by Anderson.[10] He repeatedly told them that their questions lay outside his 'area of expertise', or that his directorate did not have the information they needed, or that he did not have the necessary details (what he called the necessary 'granularity'). He told them plainly that the

Department of Health was not collecting, and was not planning to collect, data on the outcomes of the treatments given in the new centres which could be compared with NHS outcome data (and the committee heard a lot of evidence from NHS hospital doctors, who had to deal with the consequences when things went wrong in ISTCs, that there were some serious problems).[11]

While claiming that the ISTCs were 'value for money' Anderson refused point blank to give the Committee the financial information which would show whether this was true. His attitude plainly showed that he knew he enjoyed more or less total political protection. The programme was going ahead and the less MPs bothered their heads with it the better.

So the ISTC programme accomplished its primary aim of giving the private sector a foothold within the NHS, and breaking the state's effective monopoly of secondary care provision. While some of the second wave ISTC contracts were abandoned in 2007, the previous year had seen the formation of the Extended Choice Network comprising (by 2009) a total of 149 privately-owned facilities authorized to treat NHS patients. It was always anticipated that ISTCs would merge into this wider network, and that the established or 'incumbent' UK-based companies would restructure their business models to take advantage of it.

So the bridgehead had been widened. Spending on private sector acute healthcare services had doubled and NHS hospital staff were beginning to realize that more and more of them would eventually have to transfer to a private employer, on whatever terms they could get.

In 2007 Ken Anderson, his mission accomplished, left the Department to become a managing director and 'head of UK government coverage' at UBS Investment Bank in Switzerland, working with clients 'with an emphasis on health care'. Initially it was decided to replace him with Mr R. Channing Wheeler III, a vice-president in the American HMO, UnitedHealth.

Unkind critics pointed out that UnitedHealth had a record of allegations of fraudulent dealing with various branches of the US government, for which it had paid millions of dollars in reparations and fines. Moreover in 2007 Wheeler himself was under investigation, along with other senior company staff, for allegedly defrauding shareholders by backdating share options to a date when their value had fallen as low as it was ever likely to go – September 11, 2001.

Tony Blair in person defended the appointment, saying 'you should appoint the best person for the job'.[12] But within a year Mr Wheeler was gone, saving the taxpayer his large salary and his £100,000 a year tax-free housing allowance. Like Milburn, he found that he needed to spend more time with his family and also, it seems safe to assume, with his lawyers. The case was eventually settled. Wheeler and his colleagues were forced to hand back $204 million to UnitedHealth's shareholders.[13]

The Commercial Directorate was finally 'decommissioned' in 2007, although its functions were transferred to Regional Commercial Support Units, to help link private providers with NHS purchasers at the local level (rather in the way troops fan out from a bridgehead once it has been consolidated). It also bequeathed to the Department of Health a new Cooperation and Competition Panel, charged with ensuring that cooperation (to which its remit pays lip service) does not become 'anti-competitive collusion' between providers. In effect, market principles were now to govern future organizational change.

Another legacy was the Directorate's consistent record of concealing the government's true intentions, refusing to provide relevant evidence or even to collect it, and misrepresenting what there was. A particularly telling example of concealing the truth from the public was the concealment of a 'Market Sustainability Analysis' commissioned by the Directorate early in 2004. The document showed the scale of the expansion of private provision that the market saw as necessary for the ISTC programme to succeed, and made it clear that the programme was a means of levering a major domestic private health industry into existence, to take over work from the NHS. A heavily 'redacted' copy was only extracted with difficulty from the Department of Health through a Freedom of Information request in February 2005, and received little media attention.[14]

Turning NHS hospitals into businesses: 'foundation trusts' and 'payment by results'

The background to the way the marketizers tackled their second objective, of making NHS hospitals and other services into real businesses, is another case of overseas policy-shopping. In November 2001 Milburn went to Madrid, officially to recruit Spanish nurses to fill vacancies in NHS hospitals. But his opposite number in the rightwing People's Party government, health minister Celia Villalobos, had something more interesting to show him: a hospital built by the Spanish national health service, but entrusted to a private company to manage. The management enjoyed a large degree of independence from the Ministry of Health, including the freedom to set its own terms of service for doctors, nurses and other staff. Hospitals managed in this new way were called 'fundaciónes sanitarias', or 'health foundations'.

According to the Spanish government, the Alcorcon hospital, which was one of several fundaciónes set up in 1997, outperformed centrally-controlled hospitals in virtually every respect. It had shorter waiting times for serious operations and had also reduced the number of hospital beds taken up by accident and emergency patients.[15] An independent study, however, which compared the fundaciónes with traditionally managed hospitals, found that they had longer surgical waiting lists, as well as fewer staff and beds per head of population, and did fewer consultations. The head of the health services section of the main Workers' Union also accused the Alcorcon hospital of 'cherry-picking'. He said 'they send the most costly and difficult cases to the fully public hospital nearby in Mostoles. Complicated pregnancies and the badly injured from traffic accidents have all been sent there'.[16]

But Milburn liked what he was told and took the idea back to London, where it was enthusiastically picked up by the marketizers. Because NHS hospitals were already established as 'trusts' it would have been awkward to call them 'trust foundations' – in effect 'trust trusts' – and so it was decided to call them 'foundation trusts', even though this meant strictly nothing at all. The very emptiness of the label has helped to obscure their real purpose – making trusts into fully-fledged businesses.

Foundation trust hospitals in England would not be managed – at least for the time being – by private companies, but they were given the same sort of managerial independence. They would no longer be supervised by the Department of Health, but by a new independent regulator, called Monitor. Monitor would license them to provide a specified number of services each year and would have powers to ensure that they did so, while the Healthcare Commission would check their care quality standards. Otherwise they would be free to provide services as they saw fit. They would be free to borrow on the private financial market, enter into joint ventures with private companies and set their own terms of service for staff. Foundation trusts would thus resemble private companies in all but a few respects. They could only sell key assets with the permission of the Secretary of State, and would not make profits for shareholders (although Monitor would require them to make a 'prudent' surplus); also, to ensure that they remained focused on treating NHS patients, money earned from treating private patients could not exceed its existing proportion of a foundation trust's total income (the 'private patient income cap').

But the counterpart to their private sector-like freedom was that a foundation trust could go bust. Its contracts would be enforceable in the courts and it would not be able to turn to the Department of Health for help if it ran up unsustainable debts. In that event, Monitor could step in and remove the management and invite another foundation trust to take over. Or it could let the foundation trust hospital close, simply ensuring that other providers were available to fill the gap in services. In terms of incentives, this was all-important: the bottom line became the overriding measure of success.

This was not the way foundation trusts were presented to parliament and the public. Milburn told the House of Commons that the bill that introduced them was built on three principles: 'community empowerment, staff involvement and democratisation'. 'In no way', he said, could the bill 'be reasonably described as privatization, or a step in that direction'.[17]

The Department of Health also makes much of the fact that the directors of a foundation trust are not answerable to shareholders but to a board of governors which represents the 'members' of the trust – a mix of staff, patients and ex-patients, and local residents. Foundation trusts, it claims, 'have been created to devolve decision-making from central government control to local organizations and communities, so they are more responsive to the needs and wishes of their local people'.[18] But this was a fiction. When it became clear that very few local people had the time or resources, or were sufficiently interested, steps were quickly taken to ensure that the few who were actively interested could not affect policy.[19]

The reality was that foundation trust directors had to have the same freedom as private company directors. Being financially independent meant that every policy decision must be judged first and foremost on its impact on financial viability, rather than on whether, for example, it would meet the needs of this or that category of patient. The result was seen in various joint ventures which foundation trusts entered into with private companies. For example University College London Hospitals made a deal to let the biggest hospital chain owner in the US, HCA, take over its private patient unit and share the profits; while Moorfields Eye Hospital, also in London, opened a branch for private patients in Dubai. In both cases critics thought that while the deals might improve the trusts' balance sheets, they drew resources and expertise away from the treatment of NHS patients.

The aim was that by 2008 all NHS trusts should be foundation trusts. This deadline proved too tight. By early 2011 there were 125 foundation trusts, out of a possible total of over 200.[20] The Coalition government's policy is that all remaining NHS trusts are to become foundation trusts, or must have merged with a foundation trust, by 2014. At that point, virtually all NHS organizations will have to behave like private companies, or go under.

One more change was needed to prepare NHS trusts for the market: their income had to be tied more closely to their performance, as in any private business. Starting in 2004 with 'elective' procedures (such as knee replacements), and for foundation trust hospitals only, hospitals would be paid per completed treatment, and not with a lump sum for a given total of cases. This was misnamed 'payment by results' – it should have been 'payment by throughput', since whether the treatments are successful or not forms no part of the formula. It was also short of being a full market system in that price competition was ruled out. All payments were based on a national 'tariff' of fixed prices, adjusted for the seriousness of each category of case (another piece of policy-shopping, from the US). The idea was that hospitals should compete for patients on the basis of the quality of care, not price.

By the end of 2010 about 60 per cent of all NHS hospital care was being paid for on this basis (with much lower proportions for services such as mental health and ambulance services, and even less for primary care). It already meant that hospitals were more interested in some kinds of patients than others, because they are more profitable, and that the success of one hospital in attracting patients could mean destabilising the finances of another, with knock-on effects on its ability to keep staff and provide other services.

But the full significance of 'payment by results' only became fully apparent in December 2010 when the Coalition government let it be known that in future providers could be allowed to offer prices below the national tariff – in effect forcing others to compete on price. The beginnings of a full healthcare market were thus coming into view.

And so were some of its effects. In July 2010 the government had also announced the scrapping of the private patient income 'cap'. From now on foundation trusts that are well placed to attract private patients (i.e. primarily in London and other major cities) will be free to step up their private patient intake as much as they wish, if this will bring in more money than treating NHS patients. First and second class treatment within NHS hospitals will become increasingly common. Indeed, as foundation trusts grow into increasingly auto-nomous entities, detached from any national framework and increasingly reliant on private sources of both capital and revenue, we may ask if it is still appropriate to call them NHS hospitals.

* * *

These were not Alan Milburn's only contributions to the conversion of the NHS into a healthcare market, but it was left to others to complete them. In June 2003, halfway through the negotiations over a new consultants contract (described in the next chapter), he left the government, citing family reasons. He then became a paid adviser to a clutch of private companies interested in cashing in on the marketization of the NHS: Bridgepoint Capital, a venture capital company involved in financing Alliance Medical and other firms seeking NHS business; Lloyds Pharmacy; Covidien, an American manufacturer of orthotics; and last but not least, Pepsico. Pepsico's interest in health was presumably to be allowed to go on selling as many sugar-saturated soft drinks as possible. But in 2010 the new Conservative Secretary of State, Andrew Lansley, invited Pepsico to join a 'network' of businesses to help write government policy on obesity and diet-related diseases. Who knows what Milburn's role in this will be.

Milburn's model of market-friendliness would be followed by several of his ministerial successors. He himself eventually took Blairism to its logical conclusion. After giving up his seat at the 2010 election he accepted a post as the new coalition government's 'tsar' for social mobility – something for which he had certainly demonstrated an aptitude.

3

Detaching the clinical workforce from the NHS
Consultants, GPs and community health staff

If the private sector was to take over more and more NHS work it would have to take over more and more NHS staff. Getting NHS staff used to this idea, and either tempting them or obliging them (through lack of any alternative) to accept employment with for-profit firms, was an essential step if services were going to be privatized.

So the NHS Plan called for new contracts for consultants and GPs. It didn't call for new contracts for the rest of the NHS's staff, thousands of whom had already experienced being transferred to private employers during the 1980s when Thatcher made the NHS outsource cleaning, catering, laundry and other services, Over the years 1981 to 1994 non-clinical employment in the NHS had fallen from 260,000 to 120,000, and during that time those affected got scant protection for their wages and benefits. The cost reductions achieved by outsourcing, and the profits made by the outsourcing companies, were made largely by paying workers less.[1]

But although they could be very skilled, workers in these

categories often had few formal qualifications. They were seen as replaceable, and so could be transferred to private employers compulsorily. The unions did their best to defend them, as well as those who were later affected by the transfer of portering and maintenance work to the private owners of PFI hospitals from the late 1990s onwards. 'TUPE' (Transfer of Undertakings [Protection of Employment]) regulations gave them some protection against being replaced by new workers employed on worse terms, but they had no choice about transferring.

The case was different with consultants and GPs, who could not be replaced and who enjoyed high status and were well organized. Creating conditions under which they would also have to accept working for private companies was a different matter, and from the marketizers' point of view this was a key aspect of the new contracts that were heralded in the NHS Plan.

The curious incident of the new consultants' contract

As regards consultants, the NHS Plan said that more of them would get the discretionary payments (usually known as 'merit awards') that substantially increase the salaries of most senior NHS consultants, but that in future such payments would depend on their demonstrating increased 'productivity', with 'proper job plans setting out their key objectives, tasks and responsibilities and when they are expected to carry out these duties', and with 'regular reviews' of their performance. In addition, newly qualified consultants would not be able to do private work for 'perhaps seven years'.[2]

What this clearly implied was that in return for more pay consultants would be tied more closely to their NHS work, as opposed to spending time treating private patients, and would be expected to conduct that work in accordance with the wishes of hospital management – in short to reduce their professional and financial independence. This proposition, which seemed to be in the spirit of the NHS's founding values but threatened to constrain consultants' private earnings, produced a predictable stand-off. In a vote held in October 2002 a new contract on these lines was accepted by consultants in Scotland and Wales, but rejected by two-thirds of those in England.

Eventually, after Milburn had threatened to impose the new terms, his successor as health secretary, John Reid, conceded most of the English consultants' demands, awarding substantial increases in pay in return for minor adjustments to their NHS workloads and conditions of work, and without the proposed ban on private practice for newly-qualified consultants. In October 2003 a narrow majority of English consultants voted to accept the revised terms. Independent observers couldn't see that much had changed, except the size of the wage bill.[3]

What made the whole episode curious was not just the way the government seemed to simply abandon its aim of making consultants more productive (from the standpoint of hospital management) – had it not really been serious about this? (And by the way, if it really wanted consultants to do less private work, why had it agreed to let them do more and more of the work carried out by ISTCs?). What was most curious of all was that one month after the English consultants had rejected the initial contract, Dr Penny Dash, one of the chief authors of the NHS Plan, wrote an article in the *Guardian* suggesting that the idea might all along have been *not* to attach consultants more closely to the NHS but on the contrary, to antagonize them into leaving it – and that this would be a 'positive' result.[4]

Before she was appointed Director of Strategy in the Department of Health in 2000 and became centrally involved in producing the NHS Plan, Dr Dash had studied business administration in the US and worked briefly for Kaiser Permanente, the largest US HMO; from 1994 until 2000 she had worked in the London office of Boston Consulting, a leading US health consultancy. Penny Dash reappears many times in the story of the plot, moving from one influential role to another in the drive towards a healthcare market. By November 2002 she had left the Department of Health to become an 'independent adviser' to the NHS and other healthcare organizations. In her *Guardian* article she now declared that the English consultants' rejection of the contract could 'have positive and far reaching implications for the way NHS care is delivered – not least because it may open the door to more private sector provision of healthcare'.

She went on to spell out various ways in which consultants might escape control by NHS managers – the very control that the NHS Plan had said was needed. Now she suggested that in reality ministers might 'want to encourage surgeons, and indeed other groups of doctors, to form their own companies (or join existing private health providers) to sell their services back into the NHS'. 'Freed from the stifling grip of the NHS', she now wrote, they might form their own companies and negotiate with the NHS to perform procedures in either NHS or private hospitals, or form businesses of their own, raising capital and investing in new technology, or joining up with suppliers of X-ray machines and scanners and offering a 'full service solution' to 'ailing' NHS hospitals.

Such a development, she suggested, could be what 'Messrs Blair and Milburn' really wanted, and she had good reason to

Numbers and earnings of the NHS workforce in England, 2010[1]

	Number	Average total earnings
Consultants	38,745	£119,800
Registrar group	38,650	£ 57,800
Other (hospital) doctors in training	14,081	
Senior house officer		£ 42,100
House officer		£ 32,200
Hospital practitioners and clinical assistants	2,625	n.a.
Other medical and dental staff	12,420	n.a.
GPs[2]	40,269	£105,300
Nurses, midwives and health visitors	351,942	£ 31,100
Nurses, midwives and health visitors (learners)	1,409	£ 19,600
Healthcare assistants and other support staff	108,999	£ 18,200
Scientific, therapeutic and technical staff	108,581	£ 32,600
Healthcare scientists	38,609	£ 30,500
Ambulance staff	23,123	£ 32,300
Administration and estates staff	239,942	£ 21,800

Adapted from The NHS Information Centre for Health and Social Care, *NHS Staff Earnings Estimates December 2010; GP Earnings and Expenses 2008/09 Final Report; NHS Hospital & Community Health Service (HCHS) monthly workforce statistics - October 2010, Provisional, Experimental Statistics.*

1 Data for all staff except GPs are for 2010: data for GPs are for 2009. All numbers are Full Time Equivalents. Average earnings of hospital doctors shown are mean levels. Data shown for all other staff are median levels (the median – the mid-point between the highest and the lowest – is considered to give a better impression of typical earnings.) The data do not include staff working for companies providing services such as hospital cleaning to the NHS.
2 The data on GP earnings do not include those GPs holding, or employed under, Alternative Provider of Medical Services (corporate-provider) contracts, or of GPs employed by PCTs. The earnings of GPs are net of the costs of running GP practices.

know. Eighteen months earlier, when she was playing a central role in the preparation of the NHS Plan, she told a reporter from her alma mater, the Stanford Business School, that as Director of Strategy she had 'an impact on the development of the crucial strategies that will guide the NHS moving forward'.[5] Her impact should no doubt be kept in proportion. But since no one in the Department of Health saw fit to contradict her it seems fair to assume that her idea of what Messrs Blair and Milburn really wanted was shared by at least some of her departmental colleagues.

At the time few consultants seem to have taken the hint. They were perhaps partly reassured by the controversy over the introduction of foundation trusts, which took place at roughly the same time as the negotiations over the consultants' contract. The government claimed that in foundation trusts, which would no longer be subject to control from Whitehall, consultants would have more power.[6] In practice this would not prove to be the case; as we saw in chapter 2, foundation trust status meant that power was even more concentrated in the hands of chief executives.

Opponents of foundation trusts also thought that because they would be free to set their own terms of employment, and because there was a shortage of consultants, they would be able to pay consultants more, and cream off the best ones from other NHS hospitals. What critics overlooked was that the big rise in spending that underpinned the NHS Plan promised to add 7,500 consultant posts, while simultaneously shifting patient care out of hospitals. By the end of the decade consultants would actually be looking at a contracting job market, with NHS foundation trusts seeking to pay less, rather than more. In January 2010 the Foundation Trust Network, representing all foundation trusts and almost all NHS hospitals hoping to become foundation trusts – 200 organizations in all – was calling for merit awards to be abolished, pay increments to be frozen for three years, and a cap on pensions for staff earning over £100,000; and simultaneously proposing that 40 per cent of acute sector activity, the main locus of consultants' work, should be transferred to primary and community care services.[7] The Network's statement added that it could not guarantee that there would be no compulsory redundancies.

The new GP contract

Destabilizing the general practitioners' relationship with the NHS took a different tack, though building from the same premise; widespread dissatisfaction among GPs with remuneration, recruitment and work levels. While the consultants' contract seemed designed to antagonize specialists, on the surface at least the new GP contract, which was signed 2002 and came into force in 2004, gave GPs everything they wanted.

The first aspect that ensured GP compliance was a bumper increase in payments to GP practices, linked largely to demonstrating performance against a set of specific standards, the so-called Quality Outcomes Framework (QOF). These proved remarkably easy to achieve. While the Department of Health thought that the average GP practice would earn 75 per cent of the points available under the new Framework, the figure attained was in fact 91 per cent in the first year following the implementation of the contract, and 95.5 per cent by 2006-07. As the Commons Public Accounts Committee said, this 'suggested that the bar was set too low and was too easy for doctors to meet.[8]

The other aspect that guaranteed GP acceptance of the new contract was that 'out-of-hours' cover (officially defined as from 6.30pm to 8.00am on weekdays plus all day and night at weekends and public holidays), which GPs traditionally had had to provide, would now be optional; and giving up responsibility for it would entail only a modest 6% loss of income. Ninety per cent of GPs promptly opted out of providing it, and nonetheless still found themselves with an average rise in take-home earnings (after meeting the costs of running their practices) of some 30% – although salaried GPs gained much less, a point not lost on the Department of Health, as it moved to expand corporate provision of GP services. The BMA saw it as a major triumph on the part of its negotiators, Drs Simon Fradd and John Chisholm.

But giving up 'out-of-hours', plus the massive increase in earnings, soon proved to be an own goal by the GPs, and served several purposes for the marketizers. It undermined the legitimacy GPs had previously enjoyed as the sole providers of primary care. Within months of the financial effects of the new contract being reported, Hewitt declared that she wished GP incomes had been capped,[9] and GPs began to be pictured as an overpaid and outmoded profession, and in particular as being unwilling to respond to changing patient needs by opening their surgeries in the evenings and on Saturdays.

This message was reiterated by the Commons Committee, the National Audit Office and the CBI. The media of course were resolutely on message and few stories about GPs would fail to mention pay and access. And it was true that GPs – at least those who were partners, as opposed to those on salary – had received a huge pay rise, and that their leaders at first resisted the demand to have their surgeries open for longer (which of course would tend to increase their operating costs, and cut into their take-home earnings as well as give them more hours of work).

But what all this failed to acknowledge was that the Department of Health had fully anticipated that 90 per cent of GPs would opt out of providing out-of-hours care.[10] The scale of the pay rise given to most GPs may have been due to incompetence on the part of the Department of Health's negotiators, as many observers believed, but the scale of the opt-out from out-of-hours provision was something the government wanted: out-of-hours provision was seen as a useful entry-point into primary care for private companies, as well as a stick to beat GPs with (allowing them to be pictured as work-shy and overpaid). Companies such as Serco and Take Care Now were quick to seize the chance.

But providing out-of-hours primary care proved harder than it looked. In many areas Serco failed to meet any of the performance criteria for responding to urgent and emergency calls, while Take Care Now faced several charges of malpractice and finally lost most of its contracts after one of its employees, a German doctor with poor English, who was also working when exhausted, killed 70 year-old David Gray with a massive drug overdose in 2008.[11] In 2009 the private sector share of out-of-hours provision was actually lower than it had been in 2003, as GPs' extended hours in the evenings and on Saturdays reduced out-of-hours demand. Public perceptions of the quality of the mainly privately-provided out-of-hours provision varies considerably from place to place, it but has been widely criticized.

The campaign against the GPs also, however, assisted the government's promotion of a new kind of primary care contract – the 'Alternative Provider Medical Services' or APMS contract – that was introduced at the same time as the new GP contract. This replaced the traditional contract with an individual GP or a group of GP partners by one with a company employing GPs on salary, and offered a more significant opening for the private sector. It allowed PCTs to commission primary care services from large private companies such as UnitedHealth and Atos Origin (both of which were controversially awarded practices in central London), as well as from 'entrepreneurial' GP consortia and social enterprises. The aim was to increase primary care provision in under-doctored areas, but also to improve efficiency through greater competition with existing practices, including by making services more accessible. The great majority of APMS contracts highlighted the fact that they would provide services 7 days a week and from 8am to 8pm.

The issue of 'extended access' came to a head in late 2007, just when the newly-appointed Minister of Health, Lord Darzi, announced plans to roll out 'polyclinics' or larger 'GP-led health centres' on a national basis, using APMS contracts. GPs found themselves vulnerable on several fronts. In cities all practices appeared threatened with being forced to move into the new centres. 'Franchise' models of primary care were proposed, with the personalized care so valued by GPs replaced by Asda, Tesco or Virgin 'brands': it was even proposed that nurses and receptionists in the Virgin centres should wear red Virgin uniforms.[12] Payments to GP practices were frozen at the 2004 level (which had proved so much higher than expected) for a third consecutive year, the Government arguing that any increase would have to be linked to extended hours of access.

While the GPs were willing to negotiate again, the Government was not. Instead it gave them two options. GP practices must either open for longer hours, or give up more than the 6 per cent originally deducted for opting out of out-of-hours cover (it had turned out to cost more like the equivalent of 13 per cent of their incomes). As expected, the BMA took the first option, and with the GPs suitably cowed the Government pressed on with successive waves of APMS contracts. It tossed the profession a bone by awarding the majority of the first wave of these contracts to 'GP-led consortia', with private companies coming second. But this was reversed in the second wave, beginning in 2009, in which companies were awarded 40 per cent of the contracts.[13]

By July 2010 227 GP surgeries and health centres in England were being run by private companies, with nine firms, including Care UK and Assura Medical (now Virgin Assura) each holding 10 or more contracts.[14] These are not all small beer. Virgin Assura now claims to have 30 partnerships with over 1500 GPs catering for over 3 million patients, while as the market expands various new outfits, such as Intrahealth, The Practice Plc, and Malling Health, are joining the ranks of corporate providers of primary care alongside multinationals such as UnitedHealth and Atos Origin.[15]

The above figure of 40 per cent may in fact mask the overall scale of private penetration of primary care. The marketizers have routinely exploited the fact that GPs are not NHS employees but independent contractors, arguing that there is therefore nothing new in corporate provision. Such blurring has become amplified, and many providers officially referred to as 'GP-led' have in reality a commercial focus, with 'profit-making intent and a traditional corporate management structure'. The complex structure of ownership, where some private firms team up with groups of GPs, makes it 'difficult to track who controls the service and where public money is going'.[16]

Indeed, according to several private health industry journals, many GPs are becoming increasingly entrepreneurial in spirit, having 'seen the writing on the wall'. Notably the BMA's negotiators of the 2002 GP contract, Drs. Fradd and Chisholm, were among them. When the negotiations were over they set up a private company, Concordia Health, and rapidly secured several APMS contracts. All of them include offering extended opening hours.

Ms Hewitt and community health services

A very large portion of people's healthcare needs is met by community health staff, who number 250,000 in England alone – health visitors, district and community nurses, physiotherapists, speech therapists, occupational therapists, podiatrists and others, caring for a vast range of needs: people suffering from cancer, diabetes, strokes, the after-effects of surgery, mental health problems, pain. Health visitors work mostly with the parents of young children, the rest predominantly with people over 65, who bear most of society's burden of ill-health.

Some background is relevant here. When the NHS was set up in 1948 it would obviously have been rational for community health services to be integrated with the primary care services provided by GPs. But the fact that GPs insisted on remaining self-employed meant that they could not be put in charge of community health staff. Instead, responsibility for community health services was assigned to local authorities, and later to a succession of different NHS bodies, with the result that they have always been relatively neglected – chronically understaffed, suffering from skill dilution to cut costs, with inferior accommodation and IT, and no overall leadership. With the introduction of the internal market some community health trusts were established, to which community health staff were transferred, but the great majority of staff remained employed by PCTs.

By 2005 the marketizers in the Department of Health had lost patience with the slow rate of progress in reforming community health care and pushed for a market solution, and the new Secretary of State, Patricia Hewitt, agreed. She had been elected to parliament in 1997 after three years as director of research for Andersen Consulting, and the organizational problem of community health services may well have seemed to her a natural for private sector solutions. In 2005 PCTs were instructed to contract them out to other providers by the end of 2008. The result was a political uproar. Community health services might not have any medical knights to defend them, but literally millions of voters depended on them. Even the Royal College of Nursing took legal action to challenge the plan. Hewitt backtracked, in effect deferring indefinitely the date by which the outsourcing must be done.[17]

In due course community health staff were also offered a carrot: if they set themselves up as 'social enterprises' – i.e. profit-making companies, but whose profits would be devoted to social purposes – they would be given three-year contracts during which their terms of service and NHS pension rights would be preserved. But what would happen at the end of three years? Social enterprises would typically be local, relatively small, and comprising staff with very diverse skills and functions and terms of service, no experience of business and no capital. They would clearly find it difficult, to say the least, to compete successfully for a second contract, especially against large multinational companies with extensive experience of bidding, dedicated legal teams, sophisticated IT and ample access to capital, and promising to do more for less – i.e. using fewer and lower-paid staff.

Not surprisingly, by the time the Labour government finally fell few community health social enterprises had been formed. The incoming Coalition government required PCTs to stop directly employing community health staff by April 2011.By February 2011, however, it was clear that the great majority would remain in the NHS through transfers to NHS trusts and foundation trusts.[18]

* * *

Hewitt had failed to detach the bulk of the largest section of the clinical workforce, the community health staff, from the NHS, but the attachment to the NHS of both hospital doctors and GPs had been significantly weakened. When Labour ministers spoke of the 'producer interests' which stood in the way of their efforts to reform public services, doctors were among those they particularly had in mind.

Thatcher had broken the grip of consultants on hospital management, and Blair's threat to make them subject to detailed managerial control over the way they did their work with patients further weakened their allegiance to the NHS. This was even truer of GPs, whose monopoly of primary care was broken by the introduction of corporate providers of out of hours care, the new so-called GP-led health centres, and regular GP practices.

Both consultants and GPs were given substantial pay rises, for which they were then criticised on all sides. During the contract negotiations consultants felt they were being treated as enemies, and GPs felt the same over what they saw as an ultimatum over opening hours. All this led to the emergence of significant currents of opinion among both consultants and

GPs that were ready to embrace a 'new entrepreneurialism' and forge links with the private sector.

As for Hewitt, whose attitude and policies had antagonised half the staff of the Department and almost all sections of the NHS workforce, she left the cabinet in 2007 and became an adviser to the private equity company Cinven, (which had recently bought BUPA's chain of 25 private hospitals) at a salary of £60,000 for 18 days' work a year. She also became a 'special consultant' to Alliance Boots, at an annual salary of some £40,000, and a non-executive director of BT, at a salary of £60,000 (for which she would 'be expected to attend nine BT board meetings and possibly sit on committees covering remuneration and corporate and social responsibility'). In 2010 she, like Milburn, gave up politics, though not the search for private sector income, as events would show.

4

Trying to accelerate marketization
Lord Darzi, Hinchingbrooke and the debt crisis

By 2006 the basic elements of a healthcare market were in place. But there was a danger that if nothing more was done to speed things up the result could be the worst of both worlds: an NHS loaded with the costs of marketization but not offering a big enough market to attract private investment. To avoid this a more radical reorganization – or 'reconfiguration' – of the NHS was required.

Part of the solution, already sketched in the NHS Plan and tried out in the ISTC programme, was to take major components of secondary care such as diagnostics, day surgery, and the management of chronic illness, out of NHS hospitals. While there was a lot to be said for this idea, the unstated assumption attached to it was that these services would be offered to private companies to provide in other locations. This would avoid the problems that faced the two main market-oriented alternatives: first, equipping and staffing a private full-service hospital on the scale of an NHS District General Hospital, with a full range of specialties, intensive care unit, etc, which would involve heavy investment and financial risk for a private company; and second selling, not to mention giving, NHS hospitals to private companies, which would confront intense political resistance.

Another part of the solution was to hand a significant portion of primary care to for-profit providers – either GP-owned companies, or large corporations, or a mixture of the two.

Lord Darzi, polyclinics and polysystems

Two people played the key roles in trying to bring this about. One was the ubiquitous Dr Penny Dash, whom we met earlier as one of the architects of the NHS Plan, and also, apparently, of the strategy behind the government's handling of the consultants contract in 2002-03. The other was Sir Ara Darzi, Paul Hamlyn Professor of Surgery at Imperial College London, and a celebrated pioneer of 'minimally invasive' surgical techniques. In December 2006 he was asked to 'develop a strategy to meet Londoners' health needs over the next five to ten years'.

The work for his report, which was completed in June 2007, involved seven teams of specialists, plus a team of civil servants, all led by Dr Dash, and advice from no less than three American health policy consultancies.[1] The report was ready in June 2007. In the following month the incoming Brown government asked Darzi, in effect, to do the same for the whole of England. He became Baron Darzi of Denham, of Gerrards Cross, and a junior minister in the Department of Health. He finished this report in June 2008, again 'supported' by Dr Dash.

Giving marketization a veneer of clinical leadership

represented by Darzi (frequently pictured in his theatre scrubs) was shrewd: few doctors, and fewer lay commentators, were so unkind as to point out that however remarkable he might be as a surgeon, Darzi had no qualifications for developing a health strategy for Denham, let alone the whole of England. In an interview with the *Guardian* he stressed that 'being a clinician and a scientist, I only talk about things I know about'.[2] Yet within six months he felt able to conclude that what London needed was a drastic redistribution of work out of hospitals into what he called 'polyclinics', to which all or at least most GPs, and presumably numerous hospital doctors too, would relocate. Although this was not stated, the polyclinics would be largely owned and operated by private firms.

His report for London acknowledged that patients might find that their GP's surgery would then be one or two kilometres distant, but when they reached the polyclinic they would find 'large, high-quality community facilities... providing a much wider range of services... antenatal and postnatal care by midwives... healthy living information and services... community mental health services, community, social care and specialist advice, all in one place...[and] the infrastructure (such as diagnostics and consulting rooms for outpatients) to allow a shift of services out of hospital settings'.[3] Polyclinics would also be the sites of most of the new 'urgent care' centres which he thought should take over most non-life-threatening emergency work from A and E departments.

And within three months of taking on the even larger job of making recommendations for the whole of England the professor felt able to publish an interim report which recommended that polyclinics – now renamed 'GP-led health centres' – should be established nationwide, starting immediately with one for every Primary Care Trust.

In reality Darzi was closely following a script from the NHS Plan, which had sketched a glowing future in which GPs would be 'working in teams from modern multi-purpose premises alongside nurses, pharmacists, dentists, therapists, opticians, midwives and social care staff.... The consulting room will become the place where appointments for outpatients and operations are booked, test results received and more diagnosis carried out using video and tele-links to hospital specialists. An increasing number of consultants will take outpatient sessions in local primary care centres...'[4]

Once again, it is important to acknowledge that polyclinics or something like them have many advantages and have been adopted in many countries – including Cuba and the former Soviet bloc. But in Lord Darzi's scheme the idea was tied to privatization. It was clear that the development of such centres in England would, like new NHS hospitals, be privately financed, and for the most part privately owned and operated. Throughout 2007 'directors, chief executives and other senior figures from a who's who of private health providers were invited to regular off-the-record briefings, held every six weeks, to get their advice on tendering and procurement of GP-led health centres and London's polyclinics'. In December 2007 Darzi himself, having been advised that investors had become 'sceptical about markets in health', assured the last of these meetings (which Ken Anderson, now at UBS Bank, was drafted in to convene) that while the focus had shifted from ISTCs, big investment opportunities were opening up in primary care.[5]

What was really in prospect was corporate control of both primary care and a large part of existing NHS secondary care, which would be shifted into the new centres, although this was not how Darzi's report put it. His public statements were always more coded. For example his interim 2008 report for England recommended that there should be a rapid expansion of GP services in under-provided areas, 'whether they are organized on the traditional independent contractor model or by new private providers'.[6]

Along the way Lord Darzi expressed opinions on several other topics which one had not previously realized fell within the expertise of surgeons specializing in robotics, especially as regards the benefits of private sector provision. He had been 'impressed by what he had heard' of the use of individual budgets in social care (lump sums given to individuals to buy their own care, described in chapter 5) and thought they could be used for some NHS care. He declared that independent sector providers had 'helped to extend choice, add capacity and spur innovation'. They had been 'successful in introducing innovation and changing the culture of surgery'. He believed that 'the innovative practice that independent sector providers can bring will help realize dramatic improvements for patients and challenge the established ways of working among NHS organizations'.[7]

The lack of evidence for these claims – which have been examined and found wanting by, among others, the House of Commons Health Committee itself – does not seem to have troubled Lord Darzi, or Dr Dash, whose policy priorities and spin are so clearly evident throughout all the reports to which Darzi put his signature. As soon as he had signed the last one, in July 2009, he resigned, his usefulness to the government being at an end.

The fate of what were soon dubbed 'Darzi centres' is interesting. All 152 primary care trusts in England were ordered to have one up and running by April 2009, and by mid-2010 140 of them had managed to establish something that answered to the name, with 12 more due to open by the end of the year. Of the first 140, about a third were run by private companies or joint ventures with private companies.[8] But few if any of them resembled the bustling, high-tech multi-purpose facilities so glowingly advertised in Darzi's London report, complete with urgent care units and diagnostic facilities.

In practice they seem to have functioned mainly as 'walk-in' centres for predominantly young and healthy patients in cities. Virgin Health was advised that 'young male professionals were of particular interest… From a business point of view this audience are the most lucrative to recruit'. Its first planned centre, to be opened in Swindon, was identified as having 'a growing population of affluent professionals with young families' with 'about 75 per cent of the list… under 40, [and] just 4 per cent aged 60 and over'.[9] Virgin eventually pulled out of the project. In Haringey, in north London, a substantial former hospital building was demolished and replaced with a modern one for which the local PCT was committed to pay £873,000 a year for 30 years.[10] A walk-in centre was opened in it, but closed after six months. Two GP practices and some other services that already existed in the neighbourhood moved in, but nothing more.

The centres may have helped to make corporate provision of primary care seem more normal, and to prepare the way for shifting specialist care out of NHS hospitals into whatever facilities the private sector might eventually decide to set up. But their own career proved short-lived. By the end of 2010 two of them had been closed, and others (including Haringey's) faced closure, as PCTs sought to weed out uneconomic activities. Then, in February 2011, the Department of Health indicated that the whole project would be, in effect, wound up.[11]

There are probably several reasons why the polyclinic/GP-led centre project failed, well before Lansley closed it down, after so much strategic effort and spin had been invested in it. The major one was undoubtedly the onset of the credit drought resulting from the 2008 financial crisis: neither private nor government funds were now available to meet the substantial costs that Darzi's proposed reconfiguration of services would entail.[12] The term 'polyclinic', which Darzi originally used to describe the centres in London, was officially replaced by the curious term 'polysystem': i.e. keeping the idea of multiple services downloaded from hospitals, but abandoning the idea of a single centre where they would all be provided, together with all the benefits which that arrangement was supposed to confer on patients. Outside London the 'Darzi centres' established by 2010 were officially called 'GP-led health centres', perhaps to lend credibility to the claim, stressed by Darzi, that the new model would restore power to clinicians.

Another important factor was that the profitability of the first wave of the new centres seemed to depend on much higher payments per patient than ordinary GP practices received (on average three times as much, initially), which could obviously not be repeated for later ones.[13] PCTs found that they were paying up to £300,000 a year in running costs for some centres which had hardly any patients.

Worse still, from the marketizers' point of view, few GPs (and of course still fewer hospital doctors) were convinced that the change would benefit patients, and some of this scepticism had translated into anxiety among patients – all of which was of concern to the Brown government as a general election approached. GPs were not directly employed by the NHS. This gave them some leverage and few of them relocated their practices into the centres. The opposition of GPs was of particular importance to the incoming Conservative Secretary of State for Health, Andrew Lansley.

Whether the centres will one day reopen as health centres, or be put to other healthcare uses, or simply closed, will be decided by the new Commissioning Board to be established under Andrew Lansley's Health and Social Care bill.[14]

One can see this decision as purely pragmatic: the centres were not proving popular and were wasting money. Or, more likely, Lansley sees a more piecemeal, cherry-picking approach to privatizing NHS services as being more likely to be attractive to the private sector. The new legislation will permit private providers to experiment with a variety of specialist services detached from hospital settings. In contrast to his New Labour predecessors, Lansley feels no need to pretend that this will provide a rational new model of health provision, such as the Darzi centres were supposed to provide, responding more effectively to patients' needs at a time when the population is ageing and treating chronic illness becomes the priority. What is provided, and how and where, should instead be decided by market forces.

Bankruptcy as opportunity: the Hinchingbrooke story

An alternative point of entry for the private sector, which looked in some ways more promising, was to hand over the management of 'failing' NHS hospitals – meaning hospitals with large debts and inadequate incomes – to be run by private companies. In some European countries such as

Germany and Sweden publicly-owned hospitals have been sold to private companies, but in Britain few politicians would care to take responsibility for doing that. But handing over the *management* of NHS hospitals to the private sector, while keeping the ownership public – on the lines of the Spanish health foundations, in fact – might not be so difficult. If a hospital had major problems a case could be made for doing it, on the grounds that private companies could bring in superior management skills. Hinchingbrooke Hospital in Huntingdon offered a good opportunity to test the idea. It had debts equal to almost half its annual income, resulting from a series of inconsistent policy changes by the Department of Health, not from failings of its own – it was actually a low-cost operator – which it seemed to have no prospect of being able to repay.[15] In 2006 it had only been rescued by public pressure from major cuts and even possible closure. So in 2007 the government invited bids to take over its management.

Bids were made by some NHS foundation trusts, but eventually only three private companies remained in the bidding and in November 2010 it was announced that the contract had gone to one of them, Circle Health (we will meet Circle Health again in chapter 6). In 2010 KPMG's Mark Britnell (who had left the Department of Health the previous year) said he thought that Hinchingbrooke was only the first of many. He believed 20-30 more NHS hospitals could soon follow suit.[16] In fact in 2008 the Department of Health had already been expecting that over the next 20 years some 90 NHS trusts would go under.[17]

Not wasting a good crisis: David Nicholson's 'money in the tin' and Andrew Lansley's White Paper

Yet by the middle of 2010 the bidding and negotiations over Hinchingbrooke had already lasted three years. The kind of major transformation dreamed of by Tim Evans and his friends in 2000 still seemed slow in coming. Something else seemed needed to make it really start to happen. Then, in September 2007, people started queuing up to take their money out of Northern Rock. A way to accelerate progress finally looked as if it might be presenting itself in the shape of a massive economic crisis. As Obama's chief of staff, Rahm Emmanuel, said at the time, 'You never want a serious crisis to go to waste'.

By late 2008 the crisis was at its height. Lehmann Brothers was history, Northern Rock had been nationalized along with Lloyds and the Royal Bank of Scotland, and the government's debt was on course to reach 70 per cent of national income, up from around 40 per cent for most of the decade. In this situation it was obvious that public spending was going to suffer. How would this affect the NHS?

According to the Department of Health, the management consultants McKinsey (where Dr Dash was by now a partner in the company's London office) were instructed in February 2009 'to provide advice on how commissioners might achieve world class NHS productivity to inform the second year of the world class commissioning assurance system and future commissioner development. The advice from McKinsey... was provided in March 2009.' But the advice McKinsey actually gave tells a very different story.

We don't know what assumptions they were told to make but it looks as if they were told or at least encouraged to assume that NHS spending would remain constant for the next five years, and asked how productivity could be increased to cope with the rise in demand over that time. Their conclusion was that in order to find enough savings to meet the rising costs of providing health care over those years the NHS might have to shed ten per cent of its staff. When the press got hold of the report in September 2009 there was a furious reaction from the NHS workforce.

Health ministers then said that the report had been rejected, and even that it had been commissioned without their authority: the guilty party was supposed to be Mark Britnell, who was then still the Department's Director General for Commissioning and System Management.[18] Whatever the truth of this, he had by then already resigned – to join KPMG, as Head of Healthcare Europe, and later Head of Global Health (after a few months of paid 'gardening leave', a parting gift from the grateful taxpayers).[19]

But the fact was that everyone in the public sector was busy trying to work out what the crisis would mean for them, and the NHS was no exception. The McKinsey report was given one of the Department's trademark upbeat titles: 'Achieving World Class Productivity in the NHS 2009/10 – 2013/14: Detailing the Size of the Opportunity' – which in this context seemed a bit like gallows humour. Still, while the McKinsey team thought cutting up to 135,000 jobs might be unavoidable, they did explore all the theoretically possible alternative ways of saving money by making the NHS more efficient.

At any rate it was clear that the NHS Chief Executive, David Nicholson, seemed to be following the thinking of the 'rejected' McKinsey report fairly faithfully when he announced in May 2009 that the NHS 'should plan on the assumption that we will need to release unprecedented levels of efficiency savings between 2011 and 2014 – between £15 billion and £20 billion across the service [to be reached] over the three years'. He proceeded to order these savings to be made ('released'), and sooner rather than later (the term actually used was 'front-loaded').[20]

Unfortunately many if not most of the means of raising efficiency proposed by McKinsey involved reorganizing complex organizational practices, which would take time. Many of them – not least moving care out of hospitals into 'cost-efficient' settings, which McKinsey saw as promising the largest savings – required *more* spending on capital, since such settings had still to be created. The only quick or 'front-loaded' way to make savings was to cut staff; and so this was what NHS managers set about doing. All over the country NHS jobs – predictably, mostly nursing and support jobs – began to be axed, and services began to be cut back.

NHS staff protested and patients were unhappy. NHS managers watched services contract and morale decline, and registered their frustration at having no time to pursue the alternative ways of 'releasing' savings that could not be done quickly. Listening to their complaints, Nicholson finally decided to make things clear: 'I'm not interested in proposals', he said. 'I want the money in the tin; I'm counting on the money.'[21] It was no doubt a trying time for him. He will have been consoled, one imagines, by being awarded a knighthood in January 2010.

That may also have helped him come to terms with the incoming coalition government's plans to abolish Primary Care Trusts and jeopardize, probably fatally, whatever chances there might have been of realizing the efficiency savings called for by McKinsey and endorsed by him as necessary. In a speech to NHS Employers, the NHS managers' employment arm, he confessed that the experience had been emotionally upsetting, but he had finally arrived at a clear position: the essential thing was to implement government policy. 'There are people in the service who essentially hate all this [i.e. Mr Lansley's plans]', he said. 'My view is that they should go'.[22] So much for the dedication of NHS workers to universality and comprehensiveness through six decades. He added that 2,000 of them had already gone, saving the NHS £70 million a year.

In October 2010 the Coalition government announced that it would continue to raise NHS spending in real terms (based on the general consumer price index) over the next four years – the figure actually claimed was an annual rise of 0.1 per cent. As a result most people outside the NHS assumed that the cuts would now stop. But the reality was different. For one thing, the NHS was told to transfer £2.1 billion to local authorities over the next five years as part of the drive to move patients out of hospitals and into more 'cost-effective' social or community care. So the NHS budget was actually being cut. And the NHS's costs (for drugs, equipment, electricity, etc.) would go on rising faster than the general cost of living, so that even if its budget stayed more or less constant it would soon be too small to cover all the bills.

On top of this, people's healthcare needs (or 'patient demand', as today's policy-makers call patients' needs) would also go on rising as people got older, or more obese, or more depressed – and as more of them became unemployed. The economic crisis was thus also a healthcare crisis, in which drastic measures could be presented as being unavoidable, measures of 'last resort' – even if they implied the end of a high-quality health service equally available to all.

Which was pretty much what the new Secretary of State for Health, Andrew Lansley, decided to do, with proposals for yet another major NHS reorganization – a reorganization not only un-mentioned in the election campaign, but one that flatly contradicted David Cameron's election pledge not to undertake any more 'top-down reorganizations' in the NHS. Everyone noticed, of course; but the coalition's argument that the financial crisis meant that all previous bets were off proved effective – even if at first most people couldn't quite see what Lansley was driving at. All commentators agreed in calling his proposals the most important changes in the NHS since it was set up – but what exactly did the changes mean? And were they really so different from what had been covertly planned for ten years or more under New Labour?

To answer these questions we need to look first at the vision of the future healthcare system for England that the marketizers had finally evolved by the time Labour left office. Lansley's plans looked radical, but in reality they did not imply a major change of direction. The difference was mainly that what had so far been more or less successfully concealed, now came into the open.

5

The marketized NHS as New Labour policy-makers envisaged it

From 2000 until 2010 the process of 'system reform' within the NHS often looked piecemeal. But by the middle of the decade a fairly clear vision of the future healthcare market was becoming shared by policy-makers inside and outside the Department of Health. At the centre of their thinking was a particular model of 'integrated care', represented by the giant California-based HMO, Kaiser Permanente.

In January 2002 the *BMJ* had published an article which claimed that Kaiser achieved higher levels of performance than the NHS at roughly the same cost.[1] Patients enrolled in the company's 'managed care plans' were said to experience 'more comprehensive and convenient primary care services and much more rapid access to specialist services and hospital admissions' than NHS patients.

But the journal was promptly deluged with expert criticism which showed this claim to be false. Besides failing to take proper account of the many functions, from medical education to public health, that the NHS performs but which Kaiser does not, the authors' arithmetic was badly wrong. But contrary to normal practice in such cases the *BMJ* declined to publish a critical review by a group of public health academics, or to retract the article.[2]

In spite of these reservations on the part of health policy experts the government went on to invest considerable resources in promoting Kaiser as a model for the NHS to follow. Alan Milburn met with Kaiser's CEO, David Lawrence, in June 2002, accompanied by both his and Blair's special advisers, Paul Corrigan and Simon Stevens.[3] It was no doubt also relevant that the Department's Head of Strategy and Planning at the time, Penny Dash, had worked briefly for Kaiser. A series of visits to the company's Californian headquarters was organised for Department of Health policy-makers, trust executives and selected clinicians. In 2007 the Commons Health Committee went as a group to California where it 'met with academic experts, policy makers and health service providers (including Kaiser) to discuss how planning is done in a free market system and the likely shape of the future workforce'.[4]

The polyclinics and GP-led health centres envisaged by Lord Darzi, described in the previous chapter, clearly embodied many of the Kaiser model's principles, as well as offering the private sector the chance to play a central role in future NHS provision. But the implications of the HMO model, of which Kaiser is one variation, are more far-reaching than a reading of Darzi's reports indicates, and had implications for future policy that would outlive the Darzi centres.

The Kaiser model

HMOs are essentially health insurance companies that manage costs by controlling both the hospitals and other premises where care is delivered, and the clinical workforce which delivers it. Their structures vary quite widely. The Kaiser Permanente model combines all three elements – plant, workforce and insurance – in a single organization. All Kaiser doctors are shareholders or partners as well as salaried employees in the Kaiser medical groups, while the insurance arm, known as the Foundation Plan, owns and operates most of the outpatient clinics and hospitals. While the physician groups are nominally distinct, they can only work within the company's system, on the terms laid down in the Foundation Plan.

In this respect the Kaiser model does resemble the NHS (and in fact goes further, since unlike GPs in England, Kaiser's family doctors are also salaried). It is also a non-profit HMO. On the other hand it is a market-based organization, marked by a strong commercial culture. Prior to Obama's reform it could and did avoid taking on high-risk, costly patients, and was reported as cherry-picking whole communities by closing down facilities in areas of high deprivation to avoid the cost of having to provide services to uninsured victims of accidents or gunshots and other emergencies that are more common in deprived areas.

That said, the concept of integrated healthcare emphasized by Kaiser is in some obvious ways rational and desirable. Progressive reformers have long advocated similar ideas. It was even central to some pre-NHS initiatives, such as the Peckham and Finsbury Health Centres that opened in London in the 1930s. In the emerging vision of the Department of Health, however, integrated care has always been closely associated with the drive to enlarge private sector provision, and the Kaiser connection reinforced this. The competitive culture attached to integrated care in the Kaiser model, coupled with the keen interest of private providers in all integrated care initiatives, were constants, and put their stamp on official thinking about the future NHS market.

Several initiatives already taken reflect the Kaiser model. In 2003 three 'Kaiser Beacon' pilots were set up in Torbay, Northumbria, and East Birmingham. The last of these involved a 'partnership' between two PCTs and a foundation trust, and was committed to many of the Kaiser principles: integrated care; priority given to keeping patients out of hospital; active management of patients, with an emphasis on self care; clinical leadership; and extensive use of IT to underpin 'change management and patient care'.

Particular emphasis was given to the management of long-term chronic conditions, including diabetes, heart failure, and musculoskeletal disease. Patients requiring different levels of care were allocated different grades of staff, including some new, and cheaper, US imports, such as 'advanced nurse practitioners' and 'assertive case managers'. The latter were described as 'proactively engaging with a risk stratified population, providing intensive support, education for self care, coordinating care and treatment through effective multi-disciplinary working'– in effect, keeping more expensive specialist care to a minimum.[5]

Another example, resulting from a local initiative, is Principia Partners in Health, a Nottinghamshire social enterprise that looks after 115,000 patients under an APMS contract. Principia comprises 16 GP practices, with over 100 GPs, and has a staff supply agreement with Nottinghamshire County PCT for the provision of 140 nurses, therapists and managerial staff. The company combines both commissioning and provider functions, and focuses on 'practices working together to make primary care more organised, somewhat along a business model'. Although consultants do not so far appear to be involved, 'learning from Kaiser Permanente and other examples, the ambition is to develop into an NHS version of a multispecialty group practice'.[6]

A new kind of infrastructure

But a document produced in March 2006 by the NHS National Leadership Network envisaged integrated care as involving not only a shift towards more primary care-based provision, but also a radical reconfiguration of the NHS infrastructure.[7] This meant the development of new purpose-built facilities to house multidisciplinary clinical teams, and a radical reduction in the number of NHS hospitals. Smaller local hospitals would be downsized to form components of 'local urgent care networks' – closely integrated with primary care, out-of-hours care, ambulance services, social care and mental health services. Specialist care would be kept to a minimum, the aim instead being the development of what were called 'generalist specialists' who should be increasingly flexible and able to shift between different settings.

The Leadership Network did not specify who would own the resulting infrastructure, but clearly envisaged it being progressively 'decoupled' – a favourite word of the authors – from the NHS, while an expansion took place in private sector facilities. Lord Darzi's plan envisaged up to 60 per cent of NHS hospital outpatient work being transferred in this way, and Sir David Nicholson's cuts could only mean a major reduction in the number of NHS hospitals. Some of the work done previously by NHS hospitals might perhaps cease to be provided by the NHS altogether, but what was still provided would increasingly be provided in privately-owned and operated facilities.

This part of the policy-makers' vision was being anticipated in practice in a variety of ways. The ISTC programme was always intended to serve as a precursor for the much wider range of clinical activity subsequently procured under the Extended Choice Network. And all the new GP-led health centres and polyclinics have been set up under Alternative Provider Medical Services contracts, making private owner-ship the norm in the new infrastructure of primary care.

Clinician Networks

In the NHS Leadership Network's vision staff would no longer be tied to particular buildings, but would be available to work in whatever were seen as the most appropriate settings. They would increasingly be organized in independent groups, such as multidisciplinary teams, and provide their services on a contractual basis to both NHS and other providers.

Thanks to the standoff over the consultants' contract described earlier, a significant number of consultants were ready to contemplate such a move. An anaesthetist at Guy's Hospital in London said she felt that 'we are working to satisfy political objectives rather than clinical need. I find that very demoralizing'. She added that she could see the advantages of setting up a doctors 'chambers' similar to those used by barristers and selling services back to the NHS; 'I could be my own boss, work the hours I wanted to work and not be pushed about by managers or government'.[8]

A survey undertaken by *Hospital Doctor* at the time found that only 23 per cent of consultants said they were prepared to stay in the NHS till retirement age. Of the remainder, three out of ten said they planned to leave to set up private chambers.[9] And after the bruising experience of the GP contract a revived entrepreneurialism has also surfaced among a significant minority of GPs, reflected in a surge of new GP companies which are nominally led by doctors but are increasingly corporate in structure and are often joint ventures with other companies.

But the wider aim of integrated care is that clinical staff should also transcend existing institutional boundaries such as the consultant-GP divide. The National Leadership Network thought this would be achieved by 'removing key clinical staff from the direct employment of individual trusts and foundation trusts, and instead employing them via an overarching organization which would contract across traditional care boundaries to provide clinical input'.[10]

An option of this kind for both consultants and GPs wanting to leave the NHS is represented by Circle Health, the company already mentioned in chapter 4 as taking over the management of Hinchingbrooke Hospital. Circle Health is based on a model akin to the US Physician Hospital Organization, whereby large group practices and consultants own and run hospitals. With almost 1200 consultants and 600 GPs, Circle is split into three different parts. The Circle Partnership (clinicians and other staff) owns 49.9 per cent of the business; the remaining 50.1 per cent belongs to Circle International, which is owned by a group of City financial institutions; and hospital facilities are built and leased to Circle by a separate business, Health Properties Ltd. The aims of Circle are to use co-ownership to create a 'partnership of equals' and to foster a culture of clinical leadership and shared accountability; and through these to achieve improvements in patient care.[11] All staff are invited into the Partnership when they join the company, or commit a proportion of their practice to a Circle facility, and shares are available on a performance-related basis.

The chief executive of the King's Fund, Chris Ham, has praised the company as an example of how clinical leadership can thrive within a 'partnership of equals'. But since the majority shareholding belongs to Circle International, backed by private equity, clinical autonomy may not always take first place. Rather than a promise of clinical autonomy, what Circle Health seems to exemplify is the potential for a conflict between meeting health needs and meeting financial targets.

A clearer reproduction of the Kaiser model, however, was a programme of 'Integrated Care Pilots' launched by the Department of Health in April 2009. The 16 pilots selected were 'designed to explore ways in which health and social care could be provided' by looking 'beyond traditional boundaries'. New models of, for example, managing long-term conditions, could be pursued by a range of different kinds of provider, including PCTs, foundation trusts, social enterprises and private sector organizations. These organizations could 'forge new partnerships, systems and care pathways'. The previously mentioned Principia Health is one such provider. In ways akin to the HMO model the company's medical teams make contracts with local foundation trusts and PCTs. As ever the government was in a hurry and the pilot programme was rolled out several months prior to any formal evaluation.[12]

The new projects were called Integrated Care Organizations, and even the name resembles that of US Managed Care Organizations. One private company in Surrey, not part of the programme, called Integrated Health Partners, goes further and describes itself as the 'UK's first Managed Care Organization'. The company's director worked with Kaiser prior to joining McKinsey, and the management team are all former McKinsey staff.

Personal budgets for health care

The third element in the concept of integrated care promoted by the marketizers is insurance. There has been very little public discussion of insurance, for obvious political reasons: it belongs to market-based systems. In a publicly-financed and publicly-provided health service, free at the point of provision, there is nothing to insure against. But because the marketizers envisaged integrated care being provided in a market, their vision also included models of care which involved needs that could be insured for.

A leading example is the tests that are now being conducted to give patients with chronic illnesses, such as asthma and diabetes, personal budgets to spend on purchasing their care for themselves. This follows the example of the personal budgets now given to many people with disabilities to buy the personal (local authority-funded) care they need.

The government recognised that while these budgets would be for patients with predictable needs, unexpected problems could arise and the budgets might then prove inadequate. It was also pointed out that people who could afford to pay would have the option of buying more health care than their personal budgets provided for, while others could not, breaking the NHS principle of equal service free at the point of delivery. The then director of the King's Fund, Niall Dickson, said that '[if the NHS was to say] "There is £1,000 to manage your long-term condition", then if I have additional resources I could say, "Yes, I'll take that £1,000 and I'll top it up with my £500" and now I have £1,500. That would fundamentally undermine a basic principle of the NHS, which is equity of care'.[13]

But in the characteristic manner of the policy community the problem was merely noted. Dickson said that while 'caution' was required, the implementation of pilot schemes was 'commendable'. The government had in any case already awarded provisional pilot status to 68 personal health budget projects, involving 75 PCTs; and the marketizers had always seen integrated care as linked to the use of such budgets.[14] The Birmingham East and North PCT (which included one of the Kaiser Beacons) went so far as to say that 'by 2012 *all individuals* should have access to their own personal health plan and potential for personal budgets'. Such a development would 'dramatically shift care responsibility to members of the public and much of that care will be undertaken by them in their own homes'.[15] The vision of a self-paying consumer market for health care could hardly be more explicit than in this statement.

The insurance industry has been rapidly adjusting to take advantage of the opportunities this opens up to sell insurance against the risk that personal healthcare budgets will prove insufficient, beginning with insurance plans to cover the cost of certain cancer drugs which before 2010 were not provided by the NHS. Both the health insurers WPA and AXA PPP were reported to be 'enthusiastic about the potential... for the possible future expansion of such policies, whether for other medications such as those for Alzheimer's or arthritis, or for enhanced medical procedures'.[16]

Indeed, in March 2009, AXA called on PCTs to 'publish accessible information for patients on the types of treatments they might be expected to pay for themselves with "top-ups"'. The company's commercial director said 'we welcome the

Department of Health's decision to allow patients to complement their NHS treatment with privately funded care. It's a big step in the right direction of giving patients greater choice over their healthcare provision'.[17]

The insurance companies have also begun to adjust their private sector work on the lines of HMOs in the US. In 2006 Bupa Health Insurance became the first UK company to be licensed to use controversial clinical guidelines devised by the American company Milliman which they expected doctors to follow when treating patients insured with Bupa.[18] These guidelines 'cover all aspects of care from whether and what type of treatment is necessary to which type of consultant patients should see and how long they should remain in hospital'. Other private insurers are also 'increasingly using forms of "managed care" to control quality and contain their costs'.[19]

Bupa had meantime announced the creation of an ophthalmology network – a list of ophthalmologists ready to work on an agreed fee basis, who in return would get all or most of Bupa's work – and planned to roll out the same network model in other specialties, such as orthopaedics, in the ISTCs for which it had contracts (as we have seen, ISTCs depend heavily on private part-time work done by NHS consultants). The new policy meant that consultants would be paid less for simpler surgical treatments, although with the guarantee of higher volumes of work. Other insurance companies have begun to follow suit.

The insurance industry and NHS Commissioning

The reason why the development of such network arrangements in privately-insured health care is interesting is that insurers that become involved inside the NHS will naturally tend to pursue the same model there. And since 2007 insurance companies have become more and more part of the NHS landscape through their involvement in commissioning services from NHS hospitals, GPs and community care staff – influencing, if not yet actively directing, the redesign of NHS services on market-based principles.

Commissioning calls for a wide-ranging set of competences, from evaluating and redesigning services, to assessing risk, managing procurement and performance, collecting and analyzing data, securing feedback from healthcare professionals, conducting opinion surveys, and marketing. Given that Primary Care Trusts were new and relatively small, and had been subjected to frequent organizational disruptions, it was not surprising that they were seen by the marketizers as needing help from private sector expertise. So in 2007 14 companies, most of them major US and UK health insurers, were selected to assist PCTs in a Framework for Procuring External Support for Commissioners, or FESC.[20]

The assistance could range from taking on some discrete elements of the process to assuming the entire commissioning function. By mid-2010 many PCTs were working closely with FESC insurers, although no PCT had yet opted to outsource the entire task. But with the coalition government's decision to transfer commissioning responsibilities to GP Consortia, some PCTs or pathfinder consortia were bound to do that, particularly since a survey conducted in 2009 found that over 80 per cent of GPs said that they did not have the skills required.[21] The companies already closely involved in commissioning were certainly expecting this to happen. The first case arose in west London, where in

December 2010 UnitedHealth was contracted to do the commissioning for a Commissioning Consortium in Hounslow.[22]

Conclusion

By the time of the 2010 election a fairly clear picture of what the future NHS market would be like had emerged among health policy insiders. Influenced by a decade of exposure to US policy advice, and especially by the link with Kaiser Permanente, they envisaged an NHS that was already much closer to being a kitemark attached to a wide variety of provider organizations and systems than people outside the policy-making circle realized.

They imagined a radically reduced NHS hospital sector, with the surviving NHS foundation trusts focused intently on financial success. They envisaged the bulk of outpatient care being transferred out of hospitals into local, cheaper settings, which would be privately built and owned (as so many NHS hospitals already were, through PFI), or jointly owned with 'entrepreneurial' clinicians. They envisaged a growing number of the remaining NHS hospitals being run by private companies. They imagined specialist clinicians becoming increasingly self-employed, rather than working on a salary for a single foundation trust, and selling their services to a mix of public and private provider organizations.

They expected a growing proportion of patients with chronic illnesses to have fixed budgets for their care, and they accepted that top-ups, for which insurance companies would provide insurance plans, would become a normal form of co-payment, as they already were for some life-prolonging cancer drugs. They expected PCTs to be using private healthcare corporations to help them commission services in a more sophisticated way, or doing it for them, and so driving foundation trusts to become more focused on economy and directing more work to private providers. Fundamentally, they anticipated a replication of many of the structures and values of US managed care.

No one who was familiar with this imagined future could have been very surprised by the contents of Lansley's White Paper of July 2010, or the Health and Social Care Bill of January 2011. The only people likely to be surprised were the public, with whom the marketizers had chosen not to share their vision.

6

Who benefits?
The interests involved

By 2010 the private health sector in England was still very modest by international standards. Anyone who has needed health care while on holiday in Europe is likely to have become aware that much healthcare provision on the continent is private. People there are covered for most (though often not all) of the cost of care through insurance, while often having to pay fees as well (and in some countries substantial under-the-counter payments).

The contrast with the UK is striking. The private healthcare sector is still unfamiliar to anyone who doesn't have private medical insurance. But it is no longer confined to a small niche of expensive hospital treatments for purely private patients. It has been growing fast, and is increasingly confident that it is on the brink of a dramatic expansion of scale and power. Government policy since 2000 has consistently aimed at producing this result. Mr Lansley's plan, if successful, is set to complete the process, finally setting free a market dynamic that will transform the publicly-provided health service built up over the decades since 1948 into a two- or three-tier market system in which private health companies of various kinds will make a great deal of money.

What kinds of companies are these? What do they do and

how much money do they make? What are their business strategies? What do their track records suggest they will be like when they are let loose on the development of health services in England?

Some companies specialize in just one aspect of healthcare, such as acute (hospital) care. Other firms straddle more than one sector. A good example is the South African hospital chain Netcare, which opened several Independent Sector Treatment Centres in England and then bought a large chain of private hospitals from the General Healthcare Group. Another example is UnitedHealth, which now has contracts to provide GP services in various parts of England, and other contracts to handle the purchase of both GP and hospital services on behalf of various PCTs. And some British companies, such as Care UK and Tribal, have stakes in almost every kind of healthcare provision *except* hospitals, morphing into self-styled experts in any sector that looks profitable.

Other companies have made a lot of money out of NHS IT contracts, not only in the multibillion Connecting for Health (CfH) fiasco but also in projects such as the generous contract to handle NHS statistics secured by a well-networked company called Dr Foster, and the contract to operate the computerised NHS Choices system that was awarded to the all-purpose public-sector outsourcing company Capita.

Still other firms are well-established in out-of-hours primary care. The leading UK out-of-hours company, Harmoni, for example, has annual revenues of £50 million from services supplied to the NHS. Hospital cleaning, catering and laundry services provide the so-called big seven companies (ISS Mediclean, Compass Medirest, Sodexo, Mitie, Interserve, Serco and OCS) with revenues totalling almost £2 billion a year.

And the PFI programme in healthcare has proved extremely

lucrative for a host of banks, private equity financiers, construction companies and facilities management providers. Treasury figures show that the 106 NHS PFI schemes signed by September 2009 had a total capital value of £11 billion, but ongoing payments to these companies over the next three decades will amount to another £58 billion.[1] Of this, £7.1 billion are due in the five years from 2010/11 to 2015/16, which corresponds to almost half of the savings the NHS is expected to make in this period.

This proliferation of private sector firms, new and old, reflects the sheer extent of the opportunities afforded by the government to the private sector. As Milburn's health adviser, Paul Corrigan, put it: 'The state has to actively create a market, they don't appear of their own account'.[2] Such opportunities range from bloated PFI contracts and the almost risk-free ISTC programme to the guaranteed initial volumes of work offered to companies in the Extended Choice Network of private hospitals. Even in the less immediately profitable world of primary care provision the Department of Health gives companies up to three or four times more per patient than it gives to established traditional GP practices. And as we saw in chapter 5, major insurers from both sides of the Atlantic are poised to take control of much of the overall NHS budget through the commissioning function.

Given the range of services that many of these companies provide, no neat and tidy classification is possible. What we can do is follow the marketizers' template outlined in chapter 5, of hospital providers, primary care networks, and the insurance sector, and describe some of the main companies involved in each.

Hospital providers

Five companies – Netcare, Spire, Nuffield Health, Ramsay, and HCA – dominate the UK private hospital market. The size and investment strategies of two of these, particularly as they relate to the NHS, are worth looking at. We'll also look at Circle Health, which was examined in the previous chapter.

In 2006 Netcare, a newcomer from South Africa, bought the General Healthcare Group, which included the BMI chain of 60 hospitals. By mid-2009 Netcare's hospital chain comprised some 2,700 beds, with revenues of almost £750 million for the year 2008. Netcare treats NHS patients in its BMI hospital chain as well as its three Independent Sector Treatment Centres. Until 2010, the company's investments and plans focused on supporting and widening its private provision, seeing its NHS work as 'supplementary income'. It said it would 'deliver local NHS contracts in BMI hospitals using capacity that is available only "after meeting its private patient needs"' –[3] perhaps anticipating a decline in the quality of NHS provision, resulting from government spending cuts, leading to a resurgence of the private medical insurance market.

However, prior to the 2010 general election, the company showed its hand by issuing a sort of manifesto detailing numerous ways in which it thought firms like itself could aid the NHS 'whilst also boosting their own revenues'. It called for a 'moratorium on [the government] building new hospitals unless spare independent capacity has also been looked at; allowing people to pay extra for services carried out in the private sector, rather than lose their NHS entitlement; and offering tax-relief for people who self-pay for treatment, or who have private medical insurance'.[4] Netcare's BMI hospitals group chief executive, Adrian Fawcett, said 'we want to make sure that we are at the table and have laid out some ideas as to what the real areas of debate should be'.

Among these ideas Fawcett was, however, unlikely to mention was one that had occurred to his colleagues in South Africa, where according to the authorities 'poor Brazilians and Romanians were paid $6,000 (£3,840) for their kidneys to be transplanted to wealthy Israelis'.[5] The first donors, who were also Israelis, were paid up to ten times more, before the idea of going for cheaper poor people was thought of.

Prosecutors alleged that more than 100 illegal operations were conducted at a Netcare hospital in Durban between 2001 and 2003, earning 22 million rand (£2 million) for the company, and with the knowledge of the company's chief executive – charges Netcare strongly denies. But the company has admitted receiving £342,000 from an organ trafficking syndicate for work that included the removal of kidneys from five children. A statement from the company said: 'the last of the illegal operations was performed at the end of 2003. Since then Netcare and its subsidiaries have devoted considerable time and attention to ensuring that the law, the guidelines issued by the Department of Health and Netcare's own internal guidelines are meticulously adhered to and enforced in order to ensure that the conduct of deviant employees does not again cause harm to Netcare and its stakeholders'. No illegal kidney transplants in England, then. Perhaps we should feel reassured. Unfortunately unethical behaviour by many private healthcare companies in the US (touched on below and in chapter 9) shows that it is endemic in healthcare markets.

Until 2010 Netcare saw its NHS work as providing mainly supplementary income, whereas Ramsay Healthcare has, since its entry to the UK market in 2007, been heavily reliant on

NHS work. Ramsay is now the UK's fifth largest private hospital provider (its parent company is the largest private operator in Australia), owning 23 hospitals and 11 ISTCs, with almost 1000 beds. Of the company's revenues of £265 million in 2008, 44 per cent were derived from NHS activity.

Yet Ramsay's vision for the future isn't very different from Netcare's. It sees provision of private acute care as its Premium Product, and has compared its approach to the business/economy class distinction operated by airlines, with correspondingly different levels of service and choice. Its Premium Product provides 'choice of consultant, fast access, flexible appointment times, individual pre-assessment and physiotherapy, private accommodation, gift packs and à la carte menus'.[6] Its Essential Product for NHS patients, on the other hand, offers 'allocated consultant, limited procedures and appointment times, NHS access times, group physiotherapy, shared accommodation and basic food menus'. Ramsay argues that this mixed strategy 'exposes more people to the benefits and quality of the private healthcare experience' and 'strengthens relations with NHS commissioners'.[7] What the economy-class patients thought of the catering arrangements is not recorded.

Another recent entrant to the privately-owned hospital market has been Circle Health, the company which recently won the contract to manage Hinchingbrooke hospital. The company's plans are nothing if not ambitious. In 2009 it aimed to open six new state-of-the-art facilities, from Plymouth to Edinburgh, by 2011, each costing around £50 million, and, according to its chief executive, Ali Parsa, a total of up to 30 within five years. These plans have, however, been delayed, and the company's next hospital, in Reading, is not now due to open until 2012.

So far the private equity market has been providing the bulk of the company's finance, and in 2009 some commentators claimed that Circle was on the point of bankruptcy. But Parsa, a former Goldman Sachs trader, says that the necessary capital for the building programme is always on tap. Indeed the company's latest accounts showed an 80 per cent increase in revenues (to around £65 million) derived largely from its first full year of operating the UK's largest ISTC in Nottingham, as well as its other treatment centres in Bradford and Burton, all of which Circle bought from the US company Nation's Healthcare in mid-2007.

The rest of Circle's healthcare activities focus on private patients. Yet significant numbers of very senior government personnel were willing to put their weight behind it. In early 2010 the company's annual partnership conference and the simultaneous opening of its new £50 million hospital in Bath saw some 400 so-called opinion leaders in attendance. The guests included many names familiar from previous chapters, such as Lord Darzi, Chris Ham, Mark Britnell, senior Department of Health functionary Bob Ricketts, and McKinsey's head of healthcare in Europe, Nicolaus Henke, as well as health spokespersons from all the major parties. The conference was held in Audi's Bristol showrooms, no doubt deliberately mirroring the brand of healthcare provision Circle seeks to represent – high quality, not too ostentatious, no riff-raff.

Also in attendance was the chairman of the NHS Competition Panel, Lord Carter, who spoke of the need for massive NHS hospital closures over the next five years, which dovetailed neatly with Circle's hospital-building timescale.[8] We may well ask why these leading policy-makers were gracing the opening of a hospital whose main target was said to be to take 60 per cent of the Bristol market for private healthcare.[9]

The 'Kaisers' of primary care

As we saw in chapter 5, the consensus among market-orientated policy-makers is that human and physical resources need to be transferred from hospital settings to primary and even at-home care, and by 2010 the market for these had begun to assume some shape. Most of the recent arrivals on the English private healthcare scene describe themselves as GP-led, but, as we have seen, this often misrepresents their corporate nature. While some of the companies were originally set up by GPs in order to bid for local contracts against larger outfits such as Care UK and United Health, the trend is towards amalgamation between them, and the search for a wider geographical presence. A 2010 study of the 28 private companies begun by GPs and/or NHS executives for which information was available found that 18 had ambitions to expand. Similarly many joint ventures have sprung up between GPs and private companies such as Harmoni and Assura, in which ownership is divided between them.

The bulk of the contracts in primary care have so far been made under the so-called Equitable Access to Primary Medical Services initiative, which required the setting up of a GP-led health centre in every PCT and established new corporate-owned doctors' surgeries in under-doctored areas of the country. Snapping up quite a few of these contracts were relatively modest English companies such as IntraHealth, SSP Health and Malling Health, with contracts for 20, 15 and 11 GP surgeries respectively. IntraHealth, for example, which started from a base in the north-west, now has contracts in Bedfordshire, Wolverhampton and Greater Manchester. Malling Health, which began as a single surgery in Kent, has expanded in the last couple of years to take in Cambridgeshire and Somerset.

Amalgamations include the purchase in November 2010 of one of the early market leaders, Chilvers McCrea, by a rival outfit called The Practice. They already held quite a range of public sector contracts - including 23 GP LIFT schemes, six GP walk-in centres, seven contracts for prison health services and a number of outpatient clinics in areas such as ophthalmology, dermatology and sexual health.

But The Practice's chief interest is the prospect of taking on commissioning work from GPs under Mr Lansley's new Health and Social Care Bill. As the company's chief executive, Peter Watts, pointed out, while there are many GPs who want to act as commissioners, 'there are those that don't. They feel their job is to treat patients and they don't feel they have the skills to commission services, so they are asking us to do it on their behalf'.[10] The Practice expected to team up with other commissioning consortia, and while Watts acknowledged that investing on the basis of expected policy developments is a risky business, he thought developments in 2010 justified his confidence that business prospects were good.

Also seeing big opportunities in primary care and GP commissioning is Virgin Health, a fairly recent adjunct to Sir Richard Branson's conglomerate of trains, airlines and media outlets. With its usual fanfare the company held a series of marketing shows for GPs around England in 2008 with a view to opening some 50 large-scale Virgin-branded health centres, with on-site pharmacies, complementary therapy treatments and gyms. Perhaps it was the suggestion that GPs as well as nurses and receptionists working in these centres would wear Virgin's red uniform that moved a long-term member of the BMA's General Practitioners' Committee, Dr Peter Holden, to say he did not want his 'professional name attached to some hairy record shop owner'.[11] Mark Adams, the chief executive officer of Virgin Healthcare, 'sought to play down fears that the company would pose a threat to the independence of GPs, revealing they would be exempt from wearing red Virgin uniforms, unlike other staff at the surgeries'.[12] However in September 2008 the company abruptly abandoned the project, blaming poor economic conditions.

But in March 2010 Virgin bounced back into the healthcare field by purchasing one of the market leaders in corporate-provided primary care, Assura. According to *HealthInvestor*, 'most sources say that Virgin's biggest issue the first time around was working out how to make a profit from GPs without falling foul of medical regulations'. The business model was for 'patients to visit their GPs to use their free NHS Services. But they'd then stay on to use the Virgin gym or Virgin physiotherapy services elsewhere in the building. The doctors would receive a cut of the entire health centre's profits. The problem was that according to the General Medical Council's rules, this created 'a massive great conflict of interest'.[13]

How the company expected to overcome the problem is unknown, though its legal team presumably found a way.[14] But buying Assura made Virgin a significant player. Assura had formed around 30 limited liability partnerships with GP groups to 'support and maximize practice-based commissioning' and provide 'management of new care facilities in which GP practices may become providers of secondary care services, including outpatient facilities, day surgery and diagnostic services, IT infrastructure support and also property design'.[15]

The strategic role of big capital: private equity

In the following sections we look briefly at a few companies which are not necessarily big providers of NHS services, but which are playing key strategic roles in the transformation of the NHS from a public service into a healthcare market.

One category of such businesses is private equity firms. Whenever the marketization agenda has seemed to falter there have always been private equity companies to bridge the gap. Private equity companies, which came to full prominence in the 1980s, are not quoted on the stock exchange. Sometimes known as 'corporate raiders', their focus is on identifying companies from which a large medium-term profit can be made by buying, reorganizing and re-selling them. In order to bankroll their incursions into the healthcare market many companies have turned to this form of what can only be termed risky capital. Netcare's buyout of the General Healthcare Group in 2006, in what was then the biggest healthcare deal in Europe, is perhaps the prime example, although Cinven's purchase of Bupa's entire hospital portfolio in 2007, and Bridgepoint Capital's rescuing of Care UK in 2010, were also sizeable deals.

While private equity finance is both expensive and high-risk, the risk can be alleviated by being able to draw on the advice of well-placed insiders. Cinven, for example, can call on the services of Patricia Hewitt, and its portfolio of hospitals positions the company nicely for a role in the Extended Choice Network, which Hewitt herself set up. Care UK's investors' decision to sell the dominant share in their company to private equity company Bridgepoint was partly based on concerns relating to the availability of short-term profits, though presumably the longer-term optimism for growth opportunities is shared by Bridgepoint's adviser Alan Milburn.

The strategic role of big capital: framing it for the Fortune 500

Advising private equity groups interested in investing in healthcare is also part of Penny Dash's busy resumé. But while equity finance may keep market creation from stalling, a more fundamental role in market creation is that played by the huge, usually US-owned, management consultancy firms. The most important of these is McKinsey and Company, which the former management consultant David Craig says, without exaggeration, 'has gained unprecedented power over the lives of British citizens' under New Labour.[16] A major part of the company's work is helping corporations to gain access to public sectors across the globe. At the last look McKinsey's clients included more than 70 per cent of Fortune magazine's 'most-admired list', and more than 90 of the 100 'leading global corporations'. The company describes itself as follows:

> We're about world-shaping impact. We're about developing exceptional leaders. We're about trust-based relationships. We're about finding innovative solutions. We have an unparalleled depth of both functional and industry expertise as well as breadth of geographical reach. Our scale, scope and knowledge allow us to address problems no one else can.[17]

Hubristic as this sounds, as regards the company's scale and reach it is rather accurate. Whether the advice it gives is in the public interest or even good for its clients is more debatable. This became a matter of considerable public concern in relation to the UK's rail network at turn of the century, after the private company originally responsible for the track, acting on McKinsey's advice (codenamed 'Project Destiny'), abandoned a cyclical system of maintenance in favour of a policy of 'patch and mend' carried out by innumerable and often poorly-supervised sub-contractors. This led predictably to accidents, and contributed to the eventual renationalization of the network under Network Rail.[18]

From 2000 onwards the NHS in England became a key focus of McKinsey's attention, and the company became the source of a great deal of the Department of Health's thinking on system reform. After leaving the Department of Health Penny Dash worked for McKinsey as a consultant and is now a partner in its London office; and in April 2010 a former director of McKinsey, Dr David Bennett, became interim Chief Executive of Monitor – the organization which will carry out the entire regulatory function of the health service. Bennett had also previously been chief policy adviser to Tony Blair. In March 2011 he became chairman of Monitor.

In the person of Penny Dash McKinsey played a central role in Lord Darzi's 2007 proposal for the reconfiguration of London's healthcare system which aimed, among other things, to cut the staffing of non-acute services in the capital by 66 per cent, the length of GP consultations by 33 per cent, and spending on doctors by 40 per cent.[19] Dash's team was likewise behind Lord Darzi's 2008 report which extended the polyclinic model to the rest of England, and called for the expansion of commercially-run GP practices. McKinsey produced another report in 2008 for NHS London, on clinical leadership. It spoke of various 'inspirational' role models such as advocates, mentors and executive champions, who were to be the key agents in building 'a world-class healthcare system for a world-class city'. No connection was made, however, between this and the arguments of Lord Darzi's recommendations for London. The company also produced the 2009 financial analysis on which Sir David Nicholson's 'productivity savings' are based.

McKinsey's reach is particularly evident in relation to NHS commissioning, which is critical for the future of the NHS: deciding what health services are provided, as well as how, where and by whom. Such decisions are not simply practical but are framed and guided by particular belief systems. In McKinsey's case the belief is in the merits of curtailing the public sector in general, and the public provision of healthcare in particular.

Before Lansley proposed to transfer commissioning to GP consortia the two most important policy developments that gave commissioning a market-oriented character were the FESC and the so-called World Class Commissioning programme. Both of these were designed by the Department of Health in collaboration with McKinsey.

The Department asked McKinsey to assess the feasibility of market provision of commissioning –[20] i.e. of getting it done by private companies which would be invited to bid for the work. McKinsey did this by 'scoping' the capabilities and intent of the major health insurers advising on commissioning. A conflict of interest row then broke out, because McKinsey itself intended to bid for commissioning contracts against firms from which it had gained information.[21] This squabble attracted a lot of attention in healthcare industry journals, which served to deflect attention from what the policy actually implied – that is, handing the guiding role in the future evolution of the NHS to the private sector. Indeed many of the companies that complained were McKinsey clients.

The Department also asked McKinsey to draw up a 'fitness-for-purpose' review of PCTs' commissioning skills. The full range of competences which McKinsey considered necessary for reaching the status of world class was one which virtually none of the relatively newly-formed PCTs could achieve. There was an assumption in McKinsey's review that PCTs would never be able to deliver the required competencies, not least the capacity to 'stimulate the market'. In implementing the necessary changes in the PCTs, moreover, the Department of Health's Strategic Health Authorities would be able to draw on the support of a special new consortium, led by McKinsey and comprising also Ernst & Young, Kaiser Permanente, Humana and Dr Foster.[22] It was not clear, however, that this was really aimed at enabling PCTs to do the job more effectively, as opposed to giving the insurance industry greater insight into the potential NHS market.

From across the pond: UnitedHealth

A major player in the privatization of primary care and in commissioning is UnitedHealth which according to its website 'serves more than 75 million individuals, employs approximately 80,000 people and operates in all 50 states and more than 50 nations worldwide'. In 2010 UnitedHealth reported annual revenues of over $70 billion, and *Fortune* magazine ranked it as the second-largest US health insurer and number 21 of the 500 largest US corporations, based on 2009 revenues. In 2009 its CEO earned a total of $102 million.[23]

A notable feature of UnitedHealth is that it has a history of legal problems. We have already mentioned (in chapter 2) the share options scam in which the Department of Health's Channing Wheeler was involved. United's previous chief executive, Dr William McGuire, was even more deeply implicated. He was banned as a director and forced to repay $620 million to the shareholders, and barred from serving as an officer or director of a public company for ten years. He also had to pay the Securities and Exchange Commission $648 million, but was allowed to keep stock options valued at more than $800 million; his 'exit compensation' from UnitedHealth was said to be likely to be $1.1 billion.[24] The company itself, however, has also settled several cases of alleged malpractice, outlined in chapter 9.

Undeterred by this the government invited the company to play a leading role in determining how NHS services in England should be configured. As we saw in chapter 1, its first inroad was made with the Evercare programme, although this was eventually abandoned following a report on its ineffectiveness.[25] Subsequently, however, UnitedHealth was awarded contracts to run GP services in Leicester, Derby and in London. It cannot have hurt the company's efforts to place itself at the centre of the coming healthcare market in England that Simon Stevens, Tony Blair's senior health adviser from 1997 to 2004, became the company's Vice President for Global Health, and that the former editor of the *British Medical Journal*, Richard Smith, became president of UnitedHealth UK.

UnitedHealth's influence in the NHS was also enhanced by having one of its Vice Presidents, Channing Wheeler, as Ken Anderson's successor as Director General of the Commercial Directorate in the Department of Health. In his short time in the job Wheeler played a significant role in setting up the

FESC which gave major insurers a strategic foothold in redesigning the NHS. Contracts awarded under the FESC included one to UnitedHealth itself, in Northamptonshire. Another contract, which assigned responsibility for commissioning £107 million of acute and specialized services with 17 London NHS providers, was also awarded to United.[26]

The company hasn't been slow in shifting its sights to the new GP Commissioning Consortia. In October 2010, in collaboration with the pro-market National Association of Primary Care, the company published the *Essential Guide to GP Commissioning: a resource guide for professionals and managers in primary care*, to help them understand 'the fundamentals of partnership working and how it can support effective commissioning'. The CEO of the Primary Care Association said: 'working in partnership with these experts, we have been able to offer our members a summary which draws together the most practical support and advice on the immediate actions that GP teams should be taking'.[27]

Leading the way in learning from such expertise has been NHS Hounslow, which in December 2010 announced the setting up of a new referral system for patients using centralized tracking and data management designed by UnitedHealth. (Whether this is a variation on the computer system belonging to United's subsidiary Ingenix, which was at the centre of some of the company's legal troubles in New York, wasn't mentioned, though it should be pointed out that both the former CEO and a Vice President of Ingenix have since taken up directors' posts with UnitedHealth UK.)

* * *

What this chapter shows is that the process of market creation referred to by Blair's adviser, Paul Corrigan, and quoted at the outset of this chapter, has been both extensive and fast-moving. Companies of all shapes and sizes have been quick to adapt to the multiplicity of opportunities offered. Although it can appear somewhat random and piecemeal, even in primary care the trend is already towards amalgamation, wider geographical presence, and the creation of corporate management structures. Hospital groups have increasingly transformed their business models to accommodate lower-cost, higher-throughput activity, initially geared towards NHS-paid work, but increasingly also towards an anticipated growth of private work as the NHS shrinks.

And major insurers, particularly from the US, are positioning themselves to take on the NHS commissioning function, redesigning services and packaging and pricing healthcare activity into care pathways, some of which will be available on the NHS while a growing number probably won't, as the package of care available from the NHS is gradually reduced.

Alongside the experience and expertise that these corporations are said to bring to commissioning is a parallel experience of sharp practice. The rogue element that Netcare says was responsible for the kidney transplant scandal is an extreme manifestation of the market ethos in which taking opportunities to defraud the state or patients, whilst awarding outrageous sums to senior executives, all too easily becomes almost the norm. As two of the leading voices in the study of healthcare in the US, Steffie Woolhandler and David Himmelstein, ask, 'Why would anyone want to emulate the US healthcare system?' The appropriate response, they say, is not replication but quarantine.[28]

7

The health policy 'community'
How the market agenda became the only agenda

When Alan Milburn was negotiating the Concordat with the Independent Healthcare Association's Tim Evans in 2000, Blair's 'special adviser' on health was a former NHS manager called Simon Stevens. Today Stevens is in Minneapolis, as Executive Vice President, UnitedHealth Group (70 million American enrollees, $80 billion revenues), and president of its Global Health division,

UnitedHealth are as pleased with him as Milburn and Blair were. When Obama's health care reforms were before Congress, Stevens was credited with playing a key role in resisting the threat they were seen as posing to the health insurance industry. He arranged to have a large truck parked on Capitol Hill, filled with the last word in high-tech diagnostics and robotic surgery equipment. Congressmen who filed in were duly impressed. In the final version of the bill, the American health insurance industry got most of what it wanted.

In 2000 the group of insiders such as Stevens who shared,

to a greater or lesser extent, Tim Evans' faith in healthcare markets, was still fairly small. But as time went on the group expanded. Each 'reform' placed the private health industry in new positions of influence, and obliged more and more NHS staff and civil servants to come to terms with it. Step by step the marketization of the NHS advanced, and within the Department of Health and among NHS managers the idea that at least a major degree of privatization was inevitable became more and more widely accepted.

Richmond House, the Department of Health's headquarters opposite Downing Street in Whitehall, was increasingly filled with people from the private sector – not only Ken Anderson's 182 'interims' in the Commercial Directorate, but also personnel from consultancy firms of all kinds commissioned by the Department or the NHS, at a cost, in the year 2005-06 alone, of £600m.[1]

A cluster of linked organizations also developed inside and outside the NHS. Each step towards the market was consolidated by the formation of a new institution. Inside the NHS, for example, a Foundation Trust Network was formed in 2004, and an NHS Partners Network for private companies doing NHS work soon joined it. And outside – though not very far away, in practice – there was a group of well-funded think-tanks, such as the King's Fund and the Nuffield Trust; and then a wide range of interest groups, such as the PPP Forum, set up in 2001, 'the industry body for public private partnerships delivering UK infrastructure' (the largest part of which is for the NHS), and the Cambridge Health Network, set up in 2004 'to bring together leaders from the NHS and private healthcare providers'.

All these bodies, with their interlocking leaderships and memberships, and their conferences and seminars attended by ministers and senior Department officials, formed a policy-making 'community', all working with increasing confidence and common understanding to convert the NHS into a market. Only the public remained unaware.

The revolving door

The initial change in the public service outlook of the Department of Health came from importing private sector staff into key positions soon after the NHS Plan was announced, Very soon after that some senior government and civil service figures started moving into the private sector, as we saw in chapter 2.

At the Department of Health, with its huge budget (rising towards 18 per cent per cent of all government spending before the financial crisis struck), the revolving door probably revolved faster than at any other government department, except perhaps the Ministry of Defence. Coming in early were KPMG's Tim Stone, who became an adviser to the Commercial Directorate, and Sheila Masters, also from KPMG, who was put in charge of selling off land and buildings at what critics considered knock-down prices, and who later became Baroness Noakes. Deloitte's Richard Grainger was put in charge of the NHS's national IT programme, and Paul Jones came from Atos Origin (the French IT company that we saw earlier getting a contract to run a GP practice in east London) to be its chief technology officer. Penny Dash came from Boston Consulting to be the Department of Health's Head of Strategy, a role later occupied by PwC's Simon Leary.

All these people came from management consultancies. Others came from other kinds of firm, but the appeal of management consultancies to the Department of Health was that they had available staff with expertise. This was often an illusion, as former management consultant David Craig has pointed out:

> [Management] consultants are not professionals like doctors. They are not people with an interest in proffering impartial advice based on years of study and work experience. They are not trying to make you healthy. They are salespeople with sales targets to meet and bonuses to be earned. They are trying to make themselves rich. When I sold consultancy, in any month I could be in Britain acting as an expert in IT systems implementation, in Norway as an expert in oil rig construction, in France as an expert in theme park management and then back to Britain as an expert in hospital management. I never lied to my clients, but the advice that my colleagues and I gave was always and only a means to obtaining large consulting and IT systems projects so that we could meet our sales targets and earn promotions and bonuses.[2]

The results of this reliance on outside consultants can be seen in the now universally condemned PFI hospitals programme, which has made extraordinary profits for the PFI consortia and reduced many of the NHS trusts involved to near-bankruptcy, while leaving them with the obligation to go on paying for 30 years or more for buildings which experts (also from management consultancies) now say are too large. The results are also visible in the disastrous national NHS IT programme, Connecting for Health, recommended by McKinsey and managed by a consultant from Deloitte. Nine years on it is still largely inoperative, at an estimated cost to the taxpayer at least £20 billion – equivalent to all the savings that the NHS has now been told to make by 2014.[3]

Even more significant for the public interest are people who have moved in the opposite direction. Soon after they left office two successive Secretaries of State (Milburn and Hewitt) and one Minister of Health (Lord Warner) went to work for private health companies. Only slightly lower in the hierarchy were people such as Anderson and Stone and Leary (mentioned above), who came into government from the private sector and then left to put their new government connections to work back in the private sector again. And numerous well-placed career civil servants, such as Matthew Swindells, Chief Information Officer at the Department of Health, and Mark Britnell (whom we saw in chapter 4 joining KPMG), have followed suit – including, within a year, Britnell's successor as director of commissioning, Gary Belfield.

The idea that there should be a boundary between the public and private sectors, policed by ministers and civil servants as guardians of the public interest, was clearly out of fashion. As already mentioned in chapter 1, the NHS was the first and largest field for the use of the Private Finance Initiative, and the government created a big publicly-financed infrastructure to implement the policy and to promote and justify it through a huge programme of conferences and seminars, not least for Department of Health and NHS managers. One document of the Treasury Taskforce charged with implementing the PFI actually asserted an 'absolute identity of interest between the private and public sectors'.[4]

But it seems truer to say that conflicts of interest became endemic. For instance Lord Warner, after serving as a junior minister for health, took jobs advising a whole string of health-related firms:[5] Byotrol (a provider of micro biological health treatments); Apax Partners Worldwide (a private equity firm, with strong connections to the government, which has invested in health providers seeking contracts with the NHS); Deloitte (an accountancy and consultancy firm, with large revenues from government agencies); DLA Piper (a legal firm, which, like Deloitte, specialises in advising on private contracting to the public sector); and UK HealthGateway, an organization that facilitates UK market entry for medical device manufacturers ('Whatever your product – device or pharmaceutical – we employ a team of experts to guide you through the essential sales, marketing, regulatory and clinical processes and give you outstanding commercial results').

An undercover reporter posing as the representative of an overseas company interviewed Warner and concluded: 'His use [to the private sector] is his connections and the people who he knows'.[6] But the current policy-making community has a remarkably high tolerance of such behaviour. Warner remained influential inside the NHS as chairman of the north London Provider Agency, responsible for readying London's NHS hospitals to become foundation trusts.

And as we saw earlier, after quitting as Secretary of State Patricia Hewitt moved into lucrative positions with BT, Alliance Boots and Cinven – but apparently not lucrative enough. Her combined income from these positions was said to be £180,000 a year but in March 2010 she was caught by Channel 4 offering to use her contacts with ministers and civil servants, and her insight into how they work, on behalf of the imaginary clients of a fictitious US lobbying firm, for £3,000 a day. This shameless episode did not prevent her securing a rewarding position on the board of Eurotunnel a few months later.

A catalogue of less well-known people who have moved from the NHS to the private sector would take up too much space.[7] The reality was that companies which sometimes had little or no background in health care were anxious to take advantage of the opportunities being opened up in the NHS and needed to recruit knowledgeable people from inside it. It would probably be hard to find one that hasn't done so. Some of the people involved have moved back and forth between the public and private sectors, deploying their inside knowledge and contacts as profitably as possible while the transition to the market lasts.

One example among many is that of Mark Hunt, a senior adviser in the Department of Health's strategy unit. Hunt played a leading role in the production of a White Paper on Out of Hospital Care which cited Mercury Health, a division of Tribal Group, as a model of best practice in the corporate provision of primary care. Before the White Paper was published in January 2006 Hunt left the Department to become Mercury's Director of Primary Care. Then, when the White Paper he had helped to write was published, Hunt, now working for Mercury, said 'We were pleased that the Department of Health chose to highlight our role both now and in the future of the NHS'.[8] In June 2006 the company was awarded a five-year contract to run a new GP practice and walk-in centre in east London.[9]

Another case is that of an NHS manager called Tom Mann. After a stint serving as Executive Director of Inventures, a new public/private partnership enterprise mainly concerned with selling off NHS-owned land and buildings, Mann became Director of the Commercial Directorate's National Implementation Team for the ISTC programme in May 2003. But soon after, in October 2003, he left this position and in February 2004 left the civil service altogether to set up his own management consultancy, Direct Health First (DHF). He continued to work for the Directorate on a 'consultancy basis', however, until the end of May 2005, during which time the Swedish company Capio Healthcare UK was awarded a contract to run one of the largest ISTC contracts. In July 2005 Mann became the chief executive of Capio UK. (He later made an unsuccessful attempt to buy Capio, and returned to work at DHF.)[10]

Given the way the government allowed senior NHS personnel to make serious money from trading on their inside knowledge we shouldn't be surprised if many NHS managers, and even some staff, came to think that they had better start cultivating private sector options for themselves. Anyone who thought differently will have been given serious food for thought by Mr Lansley's call in July 2010 for a 45 per cent cut in management posts, and the abolition of Strategic Health Authorities and Primary Care Trusts.

Think tanks: how taxpayers help finance the corporate agenda

Very close to the Department of Health is the well-heeled world of think tanks. Some of the biggest and best-known are registered charities, which means they don't pay tax.[11]Many of them have views on health policy and publish books and research papers and hold seminars for MPs about it, but two big ones, the King's Fund and the Nuffield Trust, play a special part: between them they have more research resources than the Department of Health, and far fewer distractions. This has been especially true since 2004, when Gordon Brown cut almost 600 of the Department's 4,180 jobs. By 2006, an outside analyst noted, its 'top ranks were almost completely free of generalist civil servants' and were filled instead with NHS managers and people recruited from outside who saw their task as being to implement policy, not make it.[12] In this situation think tanks increasingly set the policy agenda.

The biggest by a long way is the King's Fund (its slogan is 'Ideas that change health care'). Originally established in 1897 to support London hospitals, the King's Fund now focuses on improving health care in England. In 2009 its income was £13.7 million. Of this £2.4 million was investment income and £1.6 million came from selling 'ideas and analysis' and 'information and support'. But the bulk – nearly £8 million – came from conferences (£1.5million) and 'developing leaders' – i.e. seminars (£6.5 million).

These too are subsidized by the taxpayer. The cost of the very high registration fees (typically £300-400 for a one-day conference or seminar) which make them so profitable (and which also exclude self-financed researchers) can be set against the tax liability of the companies whose personnel attend them, as can the cost of sponsorship. And government personnel are also strongly encouraged to attend these meetings, since it is part of the Fund's charitable mission to influence public policy and educate policy-makers. So NHS executives and Department of Health officials also attend and hear the corporate messages, with fees paid out of the health budget. In 2009 this formula allowed the King's Fund to employ some 75 professional staff, plus no less than 51 support staff.

The King's Fund insists on its independence, but its plush premises and large staff are in fact dependent on government and corporate largesse. Its board of trustees includes Simon Stevens, Julian Le Grand (successive health advisors to Tony Blair) and Penny Dash (vice-chair of the board), besides various corporate magnates. Its current Chief Executive is Chris Ham, a former director of strategy at the Department of

Health and tireless promoter of Kaiser Permanente. The most striking feature of the King's Fund is in fact the way it integrates government and corporate policy interests, and legitimizes each advance towards the market – often expressing 'concerns' and advising 'caution', but invariably ending by 'commending' it. Over the last ten years little thinking about the future of the NHS has originated far from the King's Fund. It has been consistently, if 'moderately', pro-market.

The King's Fund often collaborates with the Nuffield Trust ('for research and policy studies in health services'). The Nuffield Trust is unusual in relying primarily on a large endowment. In 2009 its investments of over £60m yielded an income of £2.38m, compared with only £900,000 of earnings from its 'charitable activities' (mostly commissioned research). In 2009 its board included Bill Moyes, the then director of Monitor (the foundation trust regulator); McKinsey's senior executive for health in Europe, Nicolaus Henke, and his McKinsey colleague Tim Kelsey; and, again, Chris Ham. Its associates include well-known pro-market academics and journalists. Not them alone: but their influence on the Trust's output is clear enough. Working with the King's Fund, and often sharing staff, the Trust has been a keen promoter of both competition and 'integration', the central elements in the marketizers' template.

Other think tanks with a significant health focus include the Reform Research Trust (usually just called Reform), which includes Doctors for Reform; Civitas; the Health Foundation; Policy Exchange; the Social Market Foundation; and the Institute for Economic Affairs.[13] Of these only the Health Foundation, chaired by the former NHS chief executive Sir Alan Langlands, is not openly committed to a healthcare market. In most cases the market commitment is clearer from their record of meetings held and publications produced (and their greater reliance on corporate donations) than from their official statements of aims. Policy Exchange, however, describes itself plainly as 'one of the UK's largest market-oriented think tanks', and the bulk of its £2.5 million income for 2008-09 was 'voluntary income', i.e. donations, which the organization spent £280,000 to raise. The sources of this income are not made public but it is not unreasonable to assume it comes largely from corporations.

On a fairly conservative estimate something like £20 million a year is being spent by think tanks to provide varying degrees of intellectual support for the drive to turn the NHS into a market system. A substantial portion of this is effectively tax-funded. The only significant work by policy researchers opposed to, or critical of, marketization has been done by UNISON, to some extent by the BMA (whose opposition, however, has been rather hesitant and qualified), and to a lesser extent UNITE, plus a range of academic experts with little or no money. Not counting the BMA, whose spending on research is not known, a generous estimate of total spending on research critical of marketization would be well under £500,000 a year.

Internal and external interest organizations

A peculiar feature of the NHS, considered as a public service, has been the existence within it of a variety of interest groups, largely financed out of the NHS budget itself. The NHS Confederation, for example, describes itself as 'the independent membership body for the full range of organizations that make up the modern NHS' – 'including ambulance trusts, acute and foundation trusts, mental health trusts and primary care trusts plus a growing number of independent healthcare organisations that deliver services on behalf of the NHS'. It claims to act in the interests both of its members and of 'patients and the public' while also 'providing an independent challenge'.

The Confederation's leadership pronounces regularly on policy issues, and gets good press coverage. While it claims to 'listen to its members' needs' and to ensure that 'their voices are heard at key stages of policy development and implementation', journalists describe it as an organisation of NHS managers. Its stance is not to criticise government policy but only to raise concerns about its feasibility, and it has evolved in accordance with the obvious 'direction of travel' being pursued by successive governments since 2000.

It has 'hosted' sub-interest groups with strong market orientations, in particular the Foundation Trust Network, which speaks for all foundation trusts and aspirant foundation trusts (which is to say, all NHS trusts), and the NHS Partners Network, which speaks for all private sector companies that are providing NHS services. Two of the Confederation's ten trustees also come from the private sector – reflecting the fact that close links between NHS organizations and the private sector are increasingly taken for granted.

A more specialized body, to which 40 NHS organizations, mainly foundation trusts, subscribe, is NHS Elect. Originally a support network for NHS elective care treatment centres, its full-time team of nine sees its role as being 'to encourage innovation and best practice and help our member organisations succeed in the evolving NHS market', by creating 'a strong culture of marketing and patient experience' and benefiting 'from new models of healthcare provision and commissioning, particularly through partnerships with other sectors'. NHS Elect's 'learning partners' include an A-list of the corporations that have been circling the NHS since the publication of the NHS Plan in 2000: Kaiser Permanente, KPMG, CHKS (a health information company now owned by Capita), and Price Waterhouse Coopers (PwC).

Formally outside the NHS, though funded by subscriptions from NHS organizations as well as from individuals, is the NHS Alliance, which describes itself as 'the only organization that brings together PCTs with practices, clinicians with managers and board members – and NHS Primary Care with its patients'. Where the Confederation claims to speak primarily for the secondary care sector, the Alliance claims to speak for primary care. It immediately threw its support behind the Lansley White Paper in July 2010, calling it a long-sought opportunity for GPs to shape the services patients want, and making no mention of the impending market.

The Alliance leadership has maintained this stance while virtually all other NHS and NHS-related bodies have expressed reservations and concerns.[14] It is hard to believe, however, that the Alliance's position actually expresses the views of most NHS community health staff or even GPs (less than a quarter of whom supported the plans).[15] It may perhaps be better understood as resembling bodies such as Nurses for Reform, described below, which claim to represent a wide base but in reality speak for a much more limited interest. The Alliance represents the 'entrepreneurial' segment of GP opinion, developed in the era of GP fundholding in the 1990s.[16]

The point about all these organizations is not that they represent and defend 'producer interests' (the public sector 'dinosaurs' who Blair said had left 'scars on his back'). If anything they provide external advocates of the market with valuable opportunities of access to senior and middle NHS management.

The health industry lobby

Unlike some other developed countries, Britain has no register of lobbyists. Firms are free to spend as much money as they like on trying to influence policy without the electorate being aware of it, and it isn't a subject on which most newspapers care to dwell. Recently, however, activists in Spinwatch and the Alliance for Transparency in Lobbying have started to lift the veil that protects the lobbying industry, and have found out quite a lot about the scale of the health industry's investment in lobbying in England, especially in recent years.[17]

The most suave end of the health industry lobby is represented by the Cambridge Health Network, set up in 2004 by (yet again) Penny Dash, in cooperation with Pam Garside, a former NHS manager and now an independent management consultant (and senior associate of the Nuffield Trust). With support from Cambridge's Judge Business School the Network aims, it says, 'to bring together leaders from the NHS and private healthcare providers (including many of the recent new entrants to the market); pharmaceutical, medical devices and biotechnology companies; retail organisations; IT, search and selection and consulting firms; think tanks and academia; and the leading financiers of health and healthcare companies'. This is done at 'private dinners with special guests and focused discussion events for sponsors, supporters and selected members', and at larger annual meetings 'hosted' by McKinsey & Co, Ernst and Young, Price Waterhouse Coopers, KPMG, the Design Council, Humana and BT Health. These events are fully paid for by a raft of very big companies – Bupa, GSK, Halliburton, Monitor, Mott Macdonald, GE, Carillion, Assura and Dell Perot Systems – most of which have major healthcare interests.[18]

Lower down the suavity scale are lobbying agencies such as Westminster Advisers and Quiller Consultants. For example the five biggest private hospital companies have formed a group for lobbying purposes called H5, which has hired the lobbying agency Westminster Advisers to press their case for greater access to the NHS budget. Another example is Capita, the outsourcing company which has 27 per cent of the UK's 'business process outsourcing' market (accounting, IT, etc) and holds extensive NHS contracts (including sole responsibility for NHS Choices, 'the digital presence of the NHS'). Capita employs Quiller Consultants, another Westminster-based company, which has strong links to the Conservatives via the far-right Centre for Policy Studies, founded by Margaret Thatcher's ideological mentor Sir Keith Joseph.

On the board of the Centre is John Nash, founder of a private equity company called Sovereign Capital, and a major donor to the Conservative Party and to Lansley's office before the 2010 election. At that time Nash was chairman of Care UK, a large residential care home owner and domiciliary care provider (the company we saw in the previous chapter being taken into care itself by another private equity firm, Bridgepoint). Sovereign Capital has investments in nine private healthcare companies.

Quite a few lobbying organisations combine lobbying with market evangelism, presenting themselves as think-tanks and sometimes even claiming to represent the sentiments and interests of the 'grassroots'. This is true of Doctors for Reform (which manages to shelter under the charitable status of Reform, described above), and Nurses for Reform, directed by Drs Helen and Tim Evans (the same Tim Evans who negotiated the concordat with Alan Milburn). Spinwatch's researcher Tamasin Cave notes that 'while NFR's links to the nursing profession are somewhat opaque, its connections to a network of pro-privatization think tanks are more apparent'.[19] These include the Adam Smith Institute, the Centre for Policy Studies, Progressive Vision, the Doctors Alliance and the Stockholm Network (which groups over 130 of them). Helen Evans has denounced the NHS as 'a Stalinist, nationalized abhorrence'.[20]

Even 2020 Health, an organization funded by big pharmaceutical companies which has campaigned to end free treatment for minor or 'lifestyle' illnesses, claims to be 'an independent, grass roots think tank', aiming to 'give back a voice and influence to those with experience in health and social care'. Its chair is Tom Sackville, a former Conservative minister, who runs the International Federation of Health Plans, representing a hundred private health insurers in 31 countries. Several of its other directors have private health sector interests. Its ties to the Conservative Party, and to Andrew Lansley in particular, are close.[21]

The labyrinthine nature of the private health lobby defies neat description. Under New Labour its impact was relatively minor, compared with the private sector's deep infiltration of the Department of Health. But the political importance of the health industry lobby in helping to end the New Labour era and opening a new phase of privatization, should not be under-estimated. It is another weapon in the private sector armoury that has helped bring the NHS as a public service close to the brink of extinction.

The Marketizer

Care UK

UnitedHealth

The King's Fund

Alan Milburn
ex-health secretary;
adviser, Bridgepoint
Capital, owners of
Care UK.

David Bennett
chair, Monitor;
ex-Blair adviser;
ex-Mckinsey.

Tony Sampson
external affairs,
United Health;
ex-Milburn private sec;
No.10 health adviser.

Simon Stevens
president global health,
UnitedHealth;
board, Kings Fund;
architect of New Labour
NHS reforms.

McKinsey

Patricia Hewitt
ex-health secretary;
adviser to Cinven,
which owns Spire.

Tony Blair

Department of Health

Spire Healthcare

Mark Britnell
head of Global
Health, KPMG;
ex-DH head of
Commissioning.

Peter Gershon
chair, GHG; ex-adviser
to Blair & Cameron.

Gary Belfield
partner, KPMG;
ex-DH acting head
of commissioning.

General Healthcare Group

KPMG

Norman Warner
ex-health minister;
ex-adviser to Apax
Partners, GHG's owners.

Matthew Swindells
Snr Exec, Cerner (US health IT giant);
ex-head of health, Tribal;
ex-NHS IT boss & adviser to Hewitt.

courtesy of Tamasin Cave at Spinwatch.org

Network

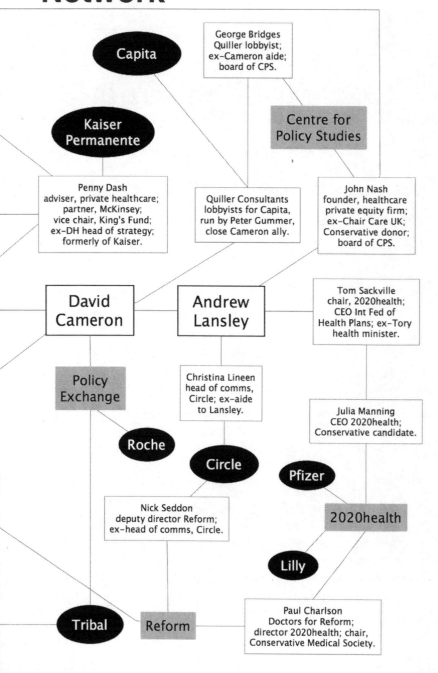

Capita

Kaiser Permanente

George Bridges
Quiller lobbyist;
ex-Cameron aide;
board of CPS.

Centre for Policy Studies

Penny Dash
adviser, private healthcare;
partner, McKinsey;
vice chair, King's Fund;
ex-DH head of strategy;
formerly of Kaiser.

Quiller Consultants
lobbyists for Capita,
run by Peter Gummer,
close Cameron ally.

John Nash
founder, healthcare
private equity firm;
ex-Chair Care UK;
Conservative donor;
board of CPS.

David Cameron

Andrew Lansley

Tom Sackville
chair, 2020health;
CEO Int Fed of
Health Plans; ex-Tory
health minister.

Policy Exchange

Christina Lineen
head of comms,
Circle; ex-aide
to Lansley.

Julia Manning
CEO 2020health;
Conservative candidate.

Roche

Circle

Pfizer

Nick Seddon
deputy director Reform;
ex-head of comms, Circle.

2020health

Lilly

Tribal **Reform**

Paul Charlson
Doctors for Reform;
director 2020health; chair,
Conservative Medical Society.

8

Casual with the truth

Lawyer: *What is the difference between a misleading
impression and a lie?*
Sir Robert Armstrong: *A lie is a straight untruth.*
Lawyer: *What is a misleading impression – a sort of bent
untruth?*
Armstrong: *As one person said, it is perhaps being
'economical with the truth'.*
(The British Cabinet Secretary cross-examined in the
Spycatcher trial in Australia, 1986)

Leaving out important facts is one form of lying. There is also
burying them – putting them in a document you are pretty
sure few people will read, or releasing it at a time when few
people will notice it. Or just keeping facts secret – for example
by declaring them 'commercially sensitive', or by deliberately
failing to collect data so that the facts remain unknown.

When none of this is possible there is always spin. Facts can
be presented as something other than what they are. Private
for-profit corporations focused on maximizing shareholder
value become 'the independent sector'. Hospital closures
become 'care in the community'. Cuts become 'productivity
savings'.

Since 2000, if not earlier, successive governments have been
pursuing a policy for the NHS that the electorate hasn't voted

for and doesn't want. In this situation the traditional civil service role of providing honest information was bound to give way to a 'corporate' culture of 'selling' the government's plans by any means possible, including all of the above. And by the early 2000s the Department of Health consisted almost wholly of people drawn from management, who readily adopted this model.[1]

Concealed entrances

With the exception of foundation trusts, none of the main steps towards the transformation of the NHS into a healthcare market down to 2010 has required legislation. They were simply announced as administrative 'reforms' in a series of documents presented to parliament, with feel-good titles that pointed anywhere but in the direction they were actually leading. It took a close reading, and an awareness of the increasingly close relationship between the Department of Health and the private health industry, to see that each of these documents concealed a new entry-point for privatization.

The *NHS Plan* of 2000 was subtitled '*a plan for investment, a plan for reform*'. Its only significant reference to the private sector was the proposed concordat, which was presented as just clearing up a tiresome history of distrust between the NHS and a potentially helpful private health sector, not as opening the door to the large-scale transfer of NHS clinical work to private companies.

The *NHS Improvement Plan* of 2004 was subtitled '*putting people at the heart of public services*'. It was actually relatively forthright about privatization, saying that PCTs would 'commission care from a wider range of providers, including independent sector organizations', and that it was expected that 'by 2008, independent sector providers will carry out up to 15% of [scheduled] procedures per annum for NHS patients'.[2] But the Improvement Plan was published in the week before parliament's summer recess, when (as it happened) all the media were focused on the adoption of the treaty for the constitution for the EU. This ensured that it attracted minimal attention. A thinly-attended House of Commons discussed it for just over an hour, and when parliament resumed in the autumn it was no longer news.

Creating a patient-led NHS (2005) said Primary Care Trusts would be required to offer patients a choice of four or five NHS providers, including any independent provider that offered treatment at NHS prices. It also talked about how NHS organizations must learn to live with risk, and how services that failed – by implication financially – would be allowed to 'exit'. This was a veiled description of how a healthcare market works: 'patient-led' was really code for 'market-based'. But the document was explicitly aimed at NHS managers, not the public. Its language was calculated not to make headlines, and didn't.

Our Health Our Care Our Say (2006) contained Hewitt's plan to make PCTs put all their provider services, which included most community health services, out to tender. It too was published in June before the recess – a favourite time for announcing controversial measures. But in the autumn, when its message had percolated out to the services involved, there was a backlash followed by a (temporary) retreat, as we saw in chapter 3.

As for Lord Darzi's final (2008) report, *High Quality Care for All*, which said all primary care would be reorganized into 'GP-led health centres', and 100 new general practices would be opened in 'under-doctored' areas, it was a notable case of being economical with the truth. It didn't mention that both measures were intended to be major openings for private providers. In fact every one of England's 152 Primary Care Trusts had been told six months earlier, in December 2007, to have a first polyclinic or health centre up and running by April 2009. When this came to light the Secretary of State, Alan Johnson, was forced to deny in parliament that the new centres were national policy and that GPs would be forced to move into them. This was closer to a straight untruth than a bent one: the private sector had been promised a substantial share of the new centres and the instructions already issued to PCTs were not revoked.[3] The report also omitted to mention something that the BMA soon learned, namely that the 100 new GP practices would also be run by companies, not traditional GP partnerships.[4]

When the real significance of each step towards the market became clear to those involved, and led to protests, the government sometimes appeared to retreat: for example with the claim that the 2009 McKinsey Report on productivity savings had been rejected, when later events clearly showed it had not been. It did the same with the initial move to make PCTs hand over both commissioning and the provision of health services to private companies. In June 2006 an invitation to tender for this work was issued, and then retracted when the scale of opposition from trade unions and others became clear. Lord Warner announced that the advertisement contained a 'drafting error': the aim, he said, was only for private companies to advise PCTs on these functions, not to take them over. But as chapter 5 shows, a takeover was always the real aim, which Lansley's plan is finally meant to achieve.[5] As soon as the clamour had died down, the advertisement was reissued with minor modification.

Another device used to head off opposition has been 'pilots'. Some of the main steps in marketization have been introduced as pilots, sometimes with a specific commitment to evaluate them before they are 'rolled out' nation-wide, which is then ignored. This tactic was eventually used to overcome opposition to involving private companies in PCT commissioning. The scheme was supposed to start in just seven 'pilot' PCTs, which the Department of Health and the Treasury could evaluate to see if it offered 'value for money'. But in March 2008, when only one pilot had even begun, let alone been evaluated, Alan Johnson announced that the scheme was to be rolled out nationally.

A final example of a concealed entry-point for private capital is lack of transparency in the bidding process. When PCTs invite bids to operate GP practices, large corporate bidders have a huge advantage over individual GPs or groups of GPs: legal teams, experience in bidding, and deep pockets (submitting a bid can easily cost upwards of £40,000). On the other hand before 2006 none of these companies had any experience in running a general practice in England. In the Derbyshire case mentioned earlier, in which Minnesota-based UnitedHealth, rather than an experienced local GP, was awarded the contract, it was clear that local knowledge and local wishes counted for little. That particular contract was overturned by the Court of Appeal on the grounds that the required local consultation had been inadequate. But in Camden, in central London, UnitedHealth went on to win three contracts against local GPs who scored higher on all the criteria listed in the invitation to tender, except cost.[6]

Secrecy and spin

The most effective way to stop people understanding what is going on is to keep it secret. For example the Department of Health has refused to release data on the runaway costs of its huge IT project, Connecting for Health (known as CfH), or the details of NHS hospital PFI contracts. The Department has also deliberately failed to collect data that would allow the results of operations done on NHS patients by private treatment centres to be compared with NHS outcome data.

There are some political costs to refusing to provide information, but the government clearly thinks they are sometimes a lesser evil. In the case of the CfH, many IT specialists who can figure out the scale of the disaster are furious, but they don't constitute an election threat. Likewise the government accepts that we will end up paying £65.1 billion for a set of PFI hospitals worth £11.3 billion, but without seeing the contracts we can't tell just how much of this is sheer rip-off.[7] And while it is a scandal that NHS patients are being referred to private treatment centres where the chances of their operations being successful are not known, the Department evidently prefers to live with it.

And what can't be concealed can be spun. The feel-good labels of 'patient-led', 'GP-led', 'community' and 'local' are endlessly replayed: Lord Darzi probably holds the record for combining the most in a single phrase: 'locally-led, patient-centred and clinically-driven'.[8] Private companies remain nearly invisible, appearing coyly in lists such as the following: 'established independent suppliers such as GPs and their teams, pharmacies and independent hospitals; other parts of the statutory sector; the voluntary sector; and new entrants from the independent, statutory or voluntary sectors'.[9]

The one word that is rarely used is 'market' – let alone 'privatization'. Instead we get 'contestability', 'plurality of provision', 'diversity of provision'. As a leading health manager said, 'Of course, contestability is simply a weasel word for competition'.[10] When the aim is to show commitment to the 'traditional' values of the NHS, GPs are cited as representing these values through the continuity of care they provide. But when GPs are seen as obstacles to marketization, we are reminded (as in the list quoted in the previous paragraph) that they are independent contractors who are in business for themselves.

Looking through the major government documents and pronouncements on the NHS over the years since 2000 is a depressing experience. Instead of reports and plans based on evidence we find tens of thousands of words aimed at securing a sort of numbed assent to proposals whose real aim is more or less camouflaged. In the last few years these reports have taken to including footnotes, giving the impression that their recommendations or plans are based on relevant evidence. But no relevant evidence is provided in support of their main aim of making health care market-driven – because the evidence shows that it makes health care more expensive and less good.

The marketizers' real attitude to evidence is like that of snake oil salesmen. If something looks as if it might help persuade, it is used; if not, it is ignored. Accuracy is of no interest. An example from Mr Lansley's White Paper shows what is involved. 'Patients want choice', it declares, and cites the 2009 British Social Attitudes survey, a well-respected source which, it says, 'shows that 95 per cent of people think that there should be at least some choice over which hospital a patient attends and what kind of treatment they receive'.

But a moment's thought raises the question – who would want no choice at all on either point? The interesting issue is whether people want choice of the kind offered by a market. On this question the British Social Attitudes survey actually tells a different story. When asked directly about choice in relation to market-based provision, it turns out that '65 per cent believe that it is more important for the NHS to ensure every patient receives the same standard of service' than that the NHS should 'meet the wishes of individual patients about how and when they are treated'. What is more, 57 per cent are opposed to private companies running NHS hospitals, compared with 22 per cent who support it. Even among those who say they want 'a great deal of choice' of hospital, more than half (54 per cent) are opposed to private companies running them.[11]

The Department of Health in fact has form on the issue of choice. In 2007 its own research arm published the results of a survey it had commissioned which found that people didn't want to have to choose a hospital when they were seriously ill, preferring their GPs to make the choice for them. Even for non-urgent surgery they only really wanted to go to the nearest hospital, unless it meant a long wait or there was a history of poor service. The Department disowned the results, saying 'the views they came up with were not those of the Department' (but, er, wasn't it the views of the *public* that were at issue?).[12]

To take one more example, among dozens. The Department was anxious to get community health workers to form 'social enterprises' as an alternative to being employed by PCTs, and said 'it is estimated that there are more than 6,000 social enterprises delivering health and social care within the NHS'.[13] For this figure it cited a *State of Social Enterprise Survey 2009*, carried out by the (non-government) Social Enterprise Coalition.[14]

This immediately seems odd: if there really were 6,000 social enterprises 'within the NHS' you would think the Department of Health would know about them itself. Odder still is the fact that the Coalition's survey could only find a total of 5,355 social enterprises in all fields in England, Scotland and Northern Ireland, so how could there be 6,000 delivering health and social care 'within the NHS'? And how could they be 'within the NHS' if they were delivering social care, which is a local authority responsibility? Moreover only six per cent of the 5,355 social enterprises in the Coalition's survey drew their funding from 'government etc', whereas any social enterprise doing NHS work would obviously be NHS-funded. In short, the 6,000 figure seems completely groundless.[15]

Consulting the public

In spite of the centrally-imposed drive to the market various bits of NHS legislation require the government 'to involve and consult patients and the public in service planning and operation, and in the development of proposals for changes'.[16] This sets up a potential contradiction: suppose people don't want the changes that the Department wants to make?

In 2003 the health minister David Lammy issued new guidance on involving patients and the public. The document's authors don't seem to have yet fully registered the contradiction. It did say NHS organizations should ask themselves, 'are people being asked to be involved in joint decision making or is this information gathering where people are asked for their views alone?' and warned against arousing expectations that couldn't be met.[17] But Mr Lammy's foreword said 'patients and the public have views to offer about the way services are operated and how they could be changed. The National Health Service must listen to this and learn from their experiences.' The guidance even added that 'a consultation allows alternative proposals to be developed'.

The contradiction involved became very clear with the public consultation on Lord Darzi's proposals for the reorganization of health care in London. The consultation, which ran for three and a half months from November 2007, produced just 4,393 individual responses from a population of 7.5 million. The questionnaire given out to the public was long, and the questions tended to ensure that the replies stacked up as desired.[18] For instance

Q: We are proposing that specialist care for children will be concentrated in hospitals with specialist child care. To what extent do you agree or disagree with this proposal?

How many people were likely to say 'No, I would prefer to send them to hospitals with no specialist child care'? What is remarkable is that 29 per cent disagreed with this particular proposal – perhaps mothers who realised it would mean long and costly journeys to one of a few hospitals that would have specialist care. A joint Oversight and Scrutiny Committee of all the London boroughs took the consultation seriously and in effect dismissed Darzi's report as full of unresolved problems.[19] The committee was impolite enough to ask the one question that had not been raised in the consultation, and that Darzi's report had studiously avoided: who was going to finance the new polyclinics? The short-run answer, as we have seen, was the private sector (to be amply repaid by the taxpayer later), but only insiders were supposed to know this.

Nothing daunted, a 'patient and public advisory group' set up by the NHS for London congratulated itself on the result of the consultation and claimed that it showed support for the Darzi plans.[20] In any case, before the London consultation was even finished PCTs had already been told to start establishing polyclinics throughout England.

Because the meaning of 'consultation' is nowhere precisely defined, the marketizers weren't much troubled by the formal obligation to consult. There was a momentary upset in 2006 when a local resident mounted a legal challenge to the decision to award the contract for a GP practice in Derbyshire, mentioned earlier, to UnitedHealth, rather than to a well-respected and popular local GP. The Court of Appeal held that the legally-required consultation had not allowed local people and patients to be involved in determining the criteria for selecting a successful bid, and ordered the contract to be re-advertised.[21] But the government subsequently issued regulations that seemed to eliminate the need to consult if the change proposed was only from public to private provision of a service, and in any case the legal costs of seeking a judicial review generally rule it out.[22] The award of GP contracts to corporate providers has gone ahead steadily, and once all NHS trusts are foundation trusts, answerable only to the regulator, the obligation to consult the public will have become meaningless.

Flak-catching

Still, the Department of Health can hardly claim to want a 'patient-centred' NHS without making at least a pretence of seeking patient and public involvement. Alan Milburn inherited a system of Community Health Councils (CHCs) set up under the Conservatives in 1974. CHCs consisted of representatives of local community organizations supported by staff to study local conditions and investigate local NHS organizations. From 1977 they also had the backing of a well-funded Association of CHCs in England and Wales.

This set-up, with its local legitimacy and resources, was clearly incompatible with turning the NHS into a market based on individual choice, rather than collective wishes. So in 2003 CHCs and their Association were abolished and replaced by Patient and Public Involvement Forums, linked to Primary Care Trusts. Unlike CHCs each Forum consisted of 7-10 individuals who happened to have put their names forward and were then appointed by the NHS Appointments Commission. They were supposed to 'gather' the views of patients and carers and represent the views of patients and the public. They had no mandate from the community to do this, and no resources to do it with.

In 2007, however, the Forums too were abolished and replaced by Local Involvement Networks or 'LINks'. These are more open-ended bodies: anyone, it seems, is welcome. This makes them potentially more representative than Patient Forums, and they have a right to enter NHS premises in search of information. But each LINk is managed by a 'host', in the shape of a local business specialising in hosting, which also holds whatever financial resources are made available. The participants in LINks have no powers beyond those of other citizens. They may provide the local NHS management with useful warnings of potential trouble, like canaries in a coal mine. Watchdogs with teeth they are not.

Dealing with dissent

Because the marketization project was pushed ahead by a Labour government it has encountered little organized national-level opposition. Unison has done most to highlight what has been happening, and commissioned some good research, but because it is linked to the Labour Party its opposition has remained ambiguous. And the BMA has been cautious and inclined to compromise, reflecting divisions of opinion within its membership.

The result has been that when individuals have spoken up about what is happening, they have had little or no organizational support. Doctors and nurses concerned about the impact of marketization on their patients have been suspended and sometimes dismissed on specious grounds, and eventually forced to accept 'gagging' clauses in costly settlement deals (with damages paid for by the NHS – i.e. by taxpayers).[23]

A revealing case that became public was that of Professor Allyson Pollock, director of the Health Policy Research Unit at University College London. In the mid-1990s she and a talented group of colleagues began examining the impact of the Private Finance Initiative on NHS hospitals. In a series of articles in the *British Medical Journal* they destroyed the economic case for the PFI.[24] Worse still, from the government's point of view, Pollock went on to challenge the marketization project more generally. She maintained close contacts with health journalists and was an excellent performer on radio and television. Each new 'reform' had journalists asking for her views.

The government's response was first to threaten and then to try to discredit her. She was replaced as a special adviser to the Commons Health Committee by a market-friendly academic. Then the head of the Department of Health's PFI Unit approached her and asked if it was 'in her career interests to brief against senior NHS officials'. Finally a back-bench MP was sent to insert some paragraphs in the Health Committee's report saying that her research unit's work showed 'a lack of sound analysis' and 'antagonistic extreme views'.[25]

This abuse of parliamentary privilege was not enough to silence Professor Pollock, but the message to any other health policy researcher who might be inclined to dissent publicly from official policy was clear: if you don't want to have your reputation trashed (not to mention being very unlikely to get any government research funding) – shut up.

9

How is the market likely to work?

Ever since the Conservatives' Health and Social Care Bill was published in January 2011, experts have been trying to work out what it is likely to mean.

The main structures are clear enough. First, PCTs will be replaced by GP Commissioning Consortia – groups of GP practices, to which all GPs must belong, and which will hold and spend the NHS budget for their patients. Second, instead of being answerable to the Secretary of State, as PCTs are, the consortia will be accountable to an independent Commissioning Board, appointed by the Secretary of State, which will determine their budgets and supervise their work. Third, all providers of secondary care – including private healthcare companies, and not just foundation trusts – will be regulated by Monitor, the independent regulator. Monitor will set the tariff of prices for NHS-paid treatments and services, including things like ambulance services. Its key mandate includes promoting competition in healthcare, drawing 'upon precedents from the utilities, rail and telecoms industries'.[1]

But how the Commissioning Board and Monitor are to use their very large discretionary powers is not specified, and so it remains to be seen how all of these components will interact in practice. For example, the government states that 'Monitor's overarching duty would be to protect and promote the interests of people who use healthcare services, by promoting competition where appropriate and through regulation where necessary'.[2] But no one knows what Monitor will consider 'appropriate' or 'necessary'.

Three issues in particular have perplexed the experts: whether the new market will encourage the development of the integrated care that was such a major goal of the marketizers under New Labour; what will be the role of patient choice; and whether there will be competition on price.

With regard to the marketizers' long-pursued theme of integrated care, soon after the Bill was published its proponents began to realise that a provider-driven market on the model of the utilities, rail and telecoms industries would not necessarily lead to integrated care. They thought that introducing competition was all right in primary care and community health services. But as Anna Dixon of the King's Fund wrote, after a discussion with Penny Dash's Cambridge Health Network, competition in specialist care needed 'careful planning', because 'the productivity challenge will require different organizations to work together', which suggested 'a more limited role for "any willing provider" markets than government policy suggests'.[3] In other words, they were starting to see that the market as Lansley envisaged it might be likely to evolve on the basis of what businessmen thought would be good for business, rather than any concern for patients.

As for patient choice, it is important for the Coalition because the White Paper of July 2010 had said 'patients will have choice of any provider, consultant-led team, choice of practice and choice of treatment'. If that was really going to be the case, and if any willing provider that met Monitor's and the Care Quality Commission's standards had the right to be listed on the Choose and Book programme, commissioning consortia would seem to have nothing to do but pay the bills submitted by the providers patients choose.

But the consortia will have tightly limited budgets and are supposed to commission what they see as innovative and efficient. How will the conflict between choice and rationing be resolved? The answer is not clear, but it looks most likely that patients will be free to choose whatever is listed on the Choose and Book list of options – provided their consortium is willing to pay for it. This is roughly the situation that already exists with PCTs – or was thought to exist, until PCTs began cutting costs by limiting GP referrals. In February 2011 the Competition and Cooperation Panel that had been bequeathed to the Department of Health by Ken Anderson's Commercial Directorate (described in chapter 2) produced an interim report that declared such restrictions anti-competitive.[4] How this is resolved should shed some interesting light on Mr Lansley's intentions on the way patient choice and consortia budget control are to be reconciled.

The question of whether providers will be allowed to compete on price, instead of only on quality, is the most important of all. The commissioning consortia, faced with budgets that won't cover everything patients need, will always be looking for ways to get providers to provide cheaper services. That is already happening with new GP contracts and outsourced community health services, and is clearly what the government expects. But what about hospital services? The Bill says that in setting the NHS tariff for services Monitor will have the power to set maximum prices, not just fixed or minimum ones. That would clearly allow competing providers to offer a lower price if they think they can still make a profit at that price.

Even most marketizers accept that price competition tends to lead to a decline in quality. In February Sir David Nicholson wrote to all NHS executives saying that there was 'no question' of price competition, apart from 'exceptional' circumstances, but as so often this proved to be at best a half-truth.[5] Just a week earlier Andrew Lansley had reminded MPs working on the Bill that only 60 per cent of hospital work was covered by the tariff, and that hospitals account for half of all NHS spending, so that 'more than half of what happens in the NHS is subject to price competition now'.[6] And David Bennett, the acting chief executive of Monitor, while expressing concern that price competition could drive down quality, nonetheless expected it to be introduced for specialist services, though 'in a limited way and very slowly'.[7] In short price competition will be fundamental to the new market. All that remains unknown is how fast it will be extended to cover specialist health care.

With price competition we can expect a decline in the quality of services, and financial crises in a good many foundation trusts as they lose revenue to private competitors. And if Monitor also allows competing providers to cherry-pick services that are relatively easy to provide such as standard operations, and the routine management of chronic illnesses, etc – and for only the least risky categories of patients, as is the case with the ISTCs, it is certain to lead to the shut-down of some hospital services, and to the closure of some hospitals.

That is because NHS hospitals currently earn money from the treatment of relatively straightforward conditions which allows them to cross-subsidize the treatment of more difficult and expensive ones. If they are left with only the latter, they will face severe financial problems. These problems will be aggravated if they are also obliged to deal with the consequences when things go wrong with the patients treated by their competitors, as has been the case up to now in relation to patients whose treatment in ISTCs has led to complications. (Indeed this also applies to patients who have been treated in private hospitals, and find themselves in need of more specialist or complicated treatment than the private hospital can provide, or more expensive treatment than their insurance will cover – since everyone has a right to NHS services.)

Monitor is supposed to ensure a 'level playing field' for all providers in the marketplace, which presumably ought to prevent this. But the chances that Monitor will police price competition across the whole of England in sufficiently close detail are not high.

And even where price competition remains excluded, private providers will still be likely to destabilize NHS hospitals if they are allowed to cherry-pick services they can provide more cheaply than hospitals, if hospitals are still required to provide a full range of services including A and E, intensive care, and so on. Private competitors will have every incentive to do so, since if they can provide a service more cheaply but are paid the same fixed price for it, they will be able to make a good profit. Again, how far Monitor allows this will be critical.

To sum up: if people were uncertain about what the Bill ultimately implied it was mainly because they had not yet fully grasped its *central aim of ultimately letting the market decide* what happens to our health services. Its key idea is that the Commissioning Board and Monitor (whose members will be appointed by the government, but not answerable to it) will oversee the transition to a full healthcare market, and then regulate it – to the extent that they think 'appropriate' or 'necessary'. And markets have their own dynamic. Once the competition genie is let out of the bottle, regulation will have at best a secondary role. The health services we will then eventually get will be what market forces produce.

The impact on quality

Commissioning consortia will be under the same pressure to cut costs as PCTs are now, and so will need to make contracts with the cheapest provider, so long as the quality is acceptable. But measuring quality is difficult, while prices are clear, and all the evidence shows that once price competition enters the picture, quality suffers. Cheaper providers are almost bound to be cutting quality somewhere, and typically on staff costs, which are the main item in all healthcare spending.

The McKinsey report on which Sir David Nicholson's cuts are based illustrates this very clearly. It called for 'efficiencies' in the shape of fewer staff doing the same or more work. For example it noted a wide variation in the number of patients district nurses see in a day, and suggested that there could be 15 per cent fewer district nurses if those who saw fewest patients in a day saw more of them. It did not enquire why some saw fewer than others – whether some worked in rural areas where patients live further apart, or whether some dealt with patients who needed more time-consuming care than others. It just recommended that the work of the district nursing service as a whole should be done with 15 per cent fewer nurses, which for an already overstretched service could only mean that fewer patients are seen, or less time is spent with them, or both – while nurses burn out and staff turnover rises.[8]

The impact of cost-cutting has already been amply demonstrated within the NHS. A notorious example is the collapse of hospital cleaning standards that occurred after private companies won contracts by cutting staff and staff wages.[9] The same effect occurred when the skill mix of nursing and care home staff – the proportion of the best-trained to the less trained – was cut to meet the high cost of leasing PFI-built hospitals, and to turn a profit in privately-owned care homes.[10] It has already happened in corporate-owned GP practices and in GP-led health centres, and is happening in the new urgent care units currently being piloted to reduce reliance on hospital A and E departments.[11] It is already evident in some outsourced community health services.

So the question for commissioning consortia will be: at what point does it become clear that the quality is not good enough? And when that point is reached, will they have enough money to allow the consortium to go back to paying more for a better service somewhere else? All the signs are that they will not.

In fact the business model of healthcare provision, depending on maximizing revenue and minimizing staff costs, is itself sufficient to destroy quality. The appalling treatment of many elderly hospital patients highlighted by the Ombudsman is a case in point.[12] Elderly patients are often admitted to hospital in a seriously ill, dehydrated and malnourished condition, with several linked problems. Getting them better takes time and attention which is in short supply when management is pressing everyone to increase *throughput*. An elderly patient who may be better but not yet ready to be discharged can quickly come to be seen not as a person in need of care, but as a 'bed-blocker', who is then consciously or unconsciously marginalized and neglected.

And the Health and Social Care Bill does not promise much enforcement of quality. In general, it stipulates that the maximum autonomy is to be given to providers, and that Monitor must regularly review the regulations to ensure that they are not 'unnecessarily burdensome'.[13] The Care Quality Commission, for its part, is authorized only to require 'essential' (i.e. minimum) standards, and has no capacity to undertake rigorous inspections on the scale required, its staff having declined from 2,900 in 2005 to 2,100 in 2010.[14] In November 2010 it abandoned routine inspections of long term care homes. [15] It relies on complaints and on whistleblowers, who have no financial incentive to reveal malpractice, and little protection when they do. Its chief executive and director explained to MPs how it relies informally on a wide range of other agencies to tell it when things are going wrong.[16] The MPs seemed remarkably unconcerned about what they were told.

Market costs

Another major downward pressure on quality is the high cost of operating a competitive market, compared with a system based on collaboration and planning. Each consortium will need to employ a team of commissioners constantly studying what providers are offering, negotiating contracts and monitoring their performance, plus bookkeepers and accountants to check and pay all the bills, lawyers to vet the contracts and conduct court cases over disputes; and a team to vet the drugs prescribed by the consortium's GPs, their referrals of patients to specialists, and the treatments proposed by the specialists. It will also need an advertising and PR department. Every hospital and chain of clinics will need the same.

In a study completed for the Department of Health in 2005 a team of researchers at York University concluded that the administrative costs of the NHS had risen from about five per cent in the mid-1970s to about 14 per cent in 2003.[17] Most of the increase was evidently due to the added costs of operating the NHS as an internal market. Since then bookkeeping and accounting and auditing costs have been further increased by the introduction of payments for each and every finished treatment in the NHS tariff (Payment by Results). The subsequent introduction of legally binding contracts for foundation trusts, and their reliance on private borrowing, will have raised costs further still.

This means that about ten per cent of the NHS's annual budget (the difference between five per cent before marketization, and over 14 per cent now), or £10 billion a year, is due to the adoption of a market system, leaving that much less to spend on health care. And with the steady extension of price competition, involving much more complex calculations of cost and benefit, administrative costs are bound to increase again. In the US it is generally reckoned that one dollar in every three spent on health care is absorbed by administrative costs. In England, with a 'single payer' (i.e. the state), they could be less, but are unlikely to be less than one pound in every four or five. Also deducted from what is spent on health care will be the dividends paid to the shareholders of private providers, and the City-level salaries paid to their senior executives.

To all this will be added the cost of insuring against the risk of overspending. The Coalition's 2010 White Paper warned: 'There will be no bail-outs for organizations which overspend public budgets', and this is going to be a chronic risk for GP Consortia. If they are too small – and early indications were that in parts of England where GPs had already started setting up 'pathfinder' consortia, most of them were much too small – they won't have a large enough 'risk pool'.[18] The beauty of a nationwide publicly-provided health service is that the risk pool consists of the whole population. Whatever the number of, say, children born with severe brain defects, or severely injured victims of traffic accidents, the high cost of looking after them is spread over England's 52 million people. Whereas if a consortium covering, say, 300,000 people finds itself responsible for an unusual cluster of such patients, the cost of caring for them will make a major hole in its limited budget. A consortium faced with that problem would have to reduce care for everyone else, or risk becoming bankrupt. Even a big consortium will need to insure against this risk, and it won't be cheap.

Fraud

A further cost arises from fraud, which is common in US health care and which seems bound to become common in England if the NHS is replaced by a market. Healthcare markets offer huge scope for fraud and other kinds of malpractice. In the US overcharging, failing to honour insurance policies, late payment of insurance claims and other kinds of malpractice are widespread. When individuals challenge the low payments insurers sometimes offer to cover insured treatments, they are frequently confronted with aggressive legal tactics, known as 'delay, diminish, deny and blame'.[19] Few can afford to fight back. When class lawsuits, or lawsuits by states, are brought against the companies involved, they are generally vigorously defended but then settled, with no admission of liability. The fines and restitutions that companies then agree to pay are seen as a cost of doing business.

The corporate culture that sustains this behaviour is driven by the overriding drive of corporate executives to raise the company's share price. The interests of patients are on the corporate agenda, but only to the extent that they affect the share price. When the two are in conflict, patients' interests come a poor second. Many of the American healthcare companies that are already involved in the NHS, and poised to play a much larger role if Mr Lansley's plans succeed, belong to that culture, and some of them have legal histories to prove it.

For example McKesson, the largest distributor of drugs in the US, and a provider of hospital equipment and IT systems, is one of the 14 companies involved in the Framework for External Support for Commissioning (FESC) outlined in chapter 5. McKesson's website says that 'Our shared values – integrity, customer-first, accountability, respect and excellence – unite us and guide us in business decisions.' But its recent history suggests otherwise. In 2009 its former chairman Charles McCall was, unusually in such cases, convicted and later sentenced to ten years in prison for fraud committed by a subsidiary of the company in 1999, for which the company had to pay shareholders $1.2 billion for losses caused by the fraud, and set aside a further $289 million to cover outstanding claims and possible tax obligations.[20] In 2009, under its next chairman, the company was forced to repay insurers and patients $350 million which it had overcharged them by manipulating the wholesale price of drugs (including drugs for cancer and other major illnesses).[21]

And then there is UnitedHealth, which has featured so extensively in the marketization story in England. In July 2002 the company was fined $1.5 million by the New York State Insurance Department. When patients were denied healthcare payments under their insurance programme the company had failed to give some of them proper notice of the right to appeal. Some months later it agreed to pay another $2.9 million to settle accusations that it had charged the US government for care to patients it falsely claimed were in nursing homes.[22] In January 2009 it agreed to pay $50 million to settle a case brought by the New York attorney general, Andrew Cuomo, for boosting profits by systematically reducing insurance repayments to patients, and in the same month paid $350 million to settle three class actions for non-payment of benefits.[23] UnitedHealth's legal problems seem never-ending. In September 2010 the State of California was seeking up to $9.9 *billion* from the company in fines for thousands of alleged legal violations, which United strenuously denied.[24]

Corporate malpractice adds significantly to the cost of health care, but more importantly it also lowers its quality, and not only because it reduces the resources available for patients. The culture that takes fraud for granted also licenses the sort of behaviour exemplified by Kaiser Permanente when it settled criminal charges for discharging a 63-year old patient and then dumping her on the street in a hospital gown and socks in a run-down area of Los Angeles. As part of the settlement Kaiser agreed to a set of rules to prevent this happening again, and to the appointment of a retired judge to monitor its observance of them. The report of the case added that Los Angeles officials said they were investigating 'more than 50 cases of dumping in downtown L.A. involving nearly a dozen hospitals'.[25]

This may sound like something that could never happen in England, but there is no reason to think so. If we accept the conversion of the NHS into a market we should expect fraud and unethical behaviour to become as usual here as it is in the US. It could actually be worse, because England lacks a political and legal culture which would offer any serious check to it. We have no law like the US False Claims Act, which since 1986 has allowed private citizens to sue on behalf of the U.S. government for alleged fraud by government contractors, and to share in any money recovered.[26]

Relative to the scale of fraud practised by healthcare companies in the US the resources of the NHS Counter Fraud and Security Management Service are modest, and in November 2010 they were scheduled to be cut. Perhaps an English equivalent of New York's energetic Attorney-General (and later Governor) Andrew Cuomo will emerge to defend the public interest, but the weak record of British governments in dealing with corporate misdeeds makes this hard to imagine.

The privatized railways effect

The combined effect of all these factors can be predicted from the experience of other regulated markets for services. There will be little to stop the cost of services rising. Monitor will have to set prices at levels which will allow private providers to make profits for shareholders (or in the case of foundation trusts, to make a surplus). But health services are far more diverse, complicated and technically complex than any other kind of service. It will be even harder for Monitor to know whether a price for a given service is necessary for providers to make a profit, than it is for the rail regulator to know what ticket prices are necessary for railway companies to make a profit. Prices will constantly be forced up.

It is also likely that private providers will eventually challenge the prices in the tariff as being insufficient, using competition law to argue that they are set to favour foundation trusts.[27] Eventually private providers may challenge the whole concept of a fixed tariff. And all providers (including foundation trusts) will stop providing services for NHS patients that are unprofitable.

The result will be a perfect storm: the withdrawal of some services, a decline in the quality of those that remain, and increases in the cost to the state which it is unable to control, leading to constant pressure to reduce the package of what is covered by the NHS. The effects already familiar from rail travel – rising ticket prices coupled with declining service, and serious compromises with safety, arising from myriad contracts and sub-contracts for which no one has overall responsibility – are all too likely to be repeated in health care.

10

What the market will mean for patients

If the Bill goes through as intended, the first thing to hit patients will be a general decline in the quality of services as the Coalition's spending cuts take effect. Then they will start to hear about the commercial companies which are increasingly deciding what sort of secondary or specialist care is available to them.

Commissioning this care – a process only made necessary, we should remember, by the purchaser-provider split as a prelude to the introduction of a full market – is technical and specialised work that few GPs can or want to do. Even those who fancy the idea of being in charge of commissioning are trained in medicine, not accounting. To call it 'GP commissioning' is misleading. The work will have to be done by the same sort of people who have been doing it for PCTs – and most likely by private sector firms, especially insurance firms with experience of competitive healthcare markets. GPs will be collaborating closely with them.

Some of these firms already have contracts to run the new commercially-owned GP practices in England and so will automatically be involved in running the GP consortia which include these practices, and in deciding how their budgets are spent. Other firms, which have been working for PCTs under the FESC scheme, are starting to work on commissioning for the new 'pathfinder' GP consortia. As already mentioned in chapter 6, one of the new pathfinder consortia, covering 57 GP practices in west London, has already signed a contract with UnitedHealth UK 'to handle all referrals, including consultant to consultant referrals, from February 2011'.[1]

Conflict of interest

Note: handle, not advise on. UnitedHealth will be controlling the referrals of all patients in Hounslow – and controlling what happens if the first consultant thinks a patient needs to be seen by a second one. The scope for conflict of interest here is large. Referring patients to be treated by a provider with which the commissioner has a financial interest may be officially banned (though monitoring this effectively seems likely to be too costly to be seriously attempted), but referring (and not referring) to other providers on a mutual back-scratching basis would seem more or less inevitable, once a large number of services are privately provided.

Will we then be sure we are being referred to the best possible secondary care for us, rather than the best for the interests of the companies involved? And how far will the kind of control the new commissioners will be exercising leave specialists free to do what they think is best for us, even if it is expensive? Will they have to get authorization from the consortium before giving the treatment? In the US, as one doctor testified before the US Congress, HMOs pay doctors doing this work a bonus related to the proportion of treatments denied.[2]

However weird it may seem, nothing in the new legislation ensures that this can't happen here. The pressures will be the same. Almost every step along the 'care pathway' will be governed by the need to turn a profit for someone: for the consortium's private sector referral managers; for the GPs and other shareholders in joint-venture centres or clinics or franchises to which patients are referred; for the doctors working in joint venture for-profit 'specialist franchises'; and for the shareholders of private hospitals and clinics treating NHS patients – and in effect also for foundation trust or social enterprise hospitals, competing to stay in business.

A quarter of GPs in England are already believed to have financial links to private healthcare companies, and the number seems likely to grow.[3] In March 2011, for example, the McKinsey-linked Integrated Health Partners mentioned in chapter 5 hit the headlines with a scheme to make some serious money. A group of GP consortia with two million patients between them would hand over their commissioning budgets to a company in which the GPs would have a 20 per cent stake. Five per cent of their combined commissioning budgets would be creamed off and booked as the firm's 'profit'. Twenty per cent of this would go to the GPs involved, and the balance (after no doubt suitably rewarding IHP's directors) would be used to float the firm on the stock market, netting almost £1 million for each GP, and raising funds to build 'healthcare facilities that would rival the NHS'.[4]

Meanwhile a new breed of doctors who combine medical and business training, called 'doctorpreneurs', is being developed by several initiatives, such as a well-networked consultancy called 'Diagnosis'. Diagnosis, which has several McKinsey-connected staff, 'offers medical students and doctors the opportunity to learn about leadership through undertaking paid projects… for a variety of clients', and through invitations to quarterly 'salons' ('a short talk followed by drinks and networking'), co-hosted by the Royal Society of Medicine.[5]

Once doctors become part of profit-making organizations the effect on the patient-doctor relationship becomes seriously corrosive. A highly-respected physician with experience of the marketization of health care in Germany sums it up as follows:

> With the increasing commercialisation of health care even well-informed patients will find themselves in a difficult situation. What is the real meaning of routine medical recommendations and information given to them in this situation? For example, 'This is not medically necessary'; or 'the risk of this intervention is in your case too high'; or 'this therapeutic intervention is not effective in your case'. Does this mean ' it is not compatible with medical knowledge and experience', or does it mean, 'it is too expensive'? How can the patient know why the doctor makes this recommendation? Is it indeed the best therapy? Will other possible treatments not be mentioned? Do such recommendations or prescriptions reflect the career or workplace interests of the physician, or perhaps the credit-worthiness of a private hospital, which determines its share price and dividend?[6]

As the medical director of Bupa has frankly acknowledged, in a healthcare market the reality is that 'conflicts of interest are everywhere'.[7] Yet the new Commissioning Consortia will have no accountability to the public for the way they spend 80 per cent of the NHS budget, but only to Monitor, which is accountable to no one at all.

The re-emergence of unequal treatment

With the removal of the cap on the amount of private patient income a foundation trust can make, anyone admitted to hospital is likely to become aware of more private patients, either in nearby private rooms, or sometimes in adjacent Private Patient Units, getting better accommodation and a lot more attention than they are. Clinical and other staff will be under pressure to divert their time and skills to private patients. The hospital they are in is also increasingly likely to be run by a private company, as Hinchingbrooke now is.

And once the political risk is judged to be low enough – that is, when we have learned to accept privatization – and when credit is more available again, privately-owned health centres of various kinds are likely to emerge after all, providing secondary care services that are currently provided by NHS hospitals. This will happen through pressure from the regulator to encourage competition, through consortia seeking ways to lower costs, and through mergers and acquisitions, as the usual process of corporate concentration leads to the swallowing up of the initial myriad small ventures, and the public monopolies that marketizers always complain about are replaced by private ones.

But given that NHS-funded work will either be based on fixed prices, or on price competition, such centres may not be the dazzlingly high-tech and comprehensive institutions painted in Lord Darzi's report. Centres of that kind will perhaps emerge where private patients constitute a high proportion of the business. Otherwise they seem more likely to just be locales to which various services have been moved, as economically as possible, from downsized or closed NHS hospitals. They will mostly be privately owned, often offering a share of the profits to the clinicians involved, and with the tendency to over-treat – especially to run unnecessary scans and tests – that is associated with profit-based healthcare everywhere, pushing up costs and increasing the pressure to reduce the list of treatments that are available free.

Community health services will also be increasingly run for profit, whether by private firms which win the contracts or by social enterprises, so long as social enterprises survive. Community health workers who have been transferred to foundation trusts will also be subject to the trusts' bottom lines. The 'five sessions and you're out' approach already applied in outsourced NHS physiotherapy, and the ever-scarcer availability of services such as podiatry (which is crucial to the ability of hundreds of thousands of mainly elderly people to get about), will become more general. And more and more people with chronic conditions will find themselves on barely adequate personal healthcare budgets, which those with sufficient means are expected to 'top up'.

Another thing patients are likely to notice is that they are more and more often invited to consider 'going private' – and as NHS services decline in quality, they will be increasingly tempted to accept. Outpatients attending NHS hospitals are already sometimes advised of nearby private services where they can get treatments more quickly. The suggestion is now increasingly apt to be made by GPs too. A majority of GPs polled in 2010 said that as a result of the 'deprioritization' (by PCTs) of treatments such as varicose veins (which can be acutely painful) they were now more likely to refer patients to the private sector.[8] Some PCTs have even deprioritized hip and knee replacements. Other treatments are being not just deprioritized but 'decommissioned' – no longer made available.

What all this adds up to is the development of a pared-down set of NHS services, beyond which patients must pay for treatment. What is available 'on the NHS' will vary, as commissioning consortia develop different priorities (not a post-code lottery but a consortium lottery). Many private sector champions argue that the NHS should introduce co-payments (fees) in the characteristic English form of 'top-ups'. A recent example is Adrian Fawcett, the chief executive of the General Healthcare Group, the largest private hospital chain in Britain. He wants 'co-paying [to be] seen as standard, so patients pay on top of their NHS care, for medicines or for their own room with extra facilities'.[9]

This seems likely to be the typical way in which fees are reintroduced, while ministers pretend that they are still defending an NHS freely available to all. Things previously taken for granted as part of the service will become extras, on the model of charges for meals on cheap airlines. To get other kinds of treatment, or more of some treatments (for example more frequent physio sessions), or to get treated sooner as waiting times lengthen again, patients will have to pay for them as top-ups – if they can afford it.

An example of what this could mean is an earlier offer made by the Queen Charlotte Hospital in London to give women the services of the same midwife throughout their pregnancy for a fee of £4,000. If you didn't pay you took your chance with a mix of whoever was available. Another NHS hospital has already charged fees to receive certain services, such as minor skin surgery, that used to be regarded as part of the NHS standard. How many finance directors of commissioning consortia will resist the temptation to try to ensure that as much cost as possible is shifted out of the consortium's budget onto patients in this way?

The chances are not good that the list of what is freely available on the NHS will improve over time. All the pressures are the other way. It is already possible for cancer patients with sufficient means to top up their NHS treatment by buying additional expensive drugs not available on the NHS. People who have been given personal budgets for NHS care for some chronic illnesses, described in chapter 5, can buy additional care from private providers if they have enough money. Many more conditions are likely to be made subject to personal budgets. Advocates of personal budgets often see maternity services as a good service to be funded in this way. These budgets too will be squeezed, creating a strong temptation for commissioners to redefine some items the budgets originally covered as extras that must be paid for.

It should be emphasized that all this has nothing whatever to do with the absolute cost of health services being 'unaffordable' or 'unsustainable', as advocates of private health care and fees always maintain. The UK still spends considerably less on health care per head than comparable EU countries. What is at issue is a choice about how a service that everyone needs should be paid for. The effect of privatizing care is to shift some of the cost from the community as a whole to individuals who have unequal abilities to pay for it. What it implies is the emergence of a three-tier healthcare system – an increasingly basic NHS service; NHS services topped up with either private services, or fee-paid additional NHS care; and fully private services.

Mr Lansley's gamble with our health

The Conservatives' drive to a full healthcare market wasn't 'a bolt from the blue', as some people pretend.[10] Virtually all of it was clearly spelled out in a Conservative Party document published by Lansley and Cameron in 2007, called 'NHS Autonomy and Accountability: Proposals for legislation'. They even called it a 'White Paper' and promised consultations on it. It is true that we were lulled into thinking there would be no major changes to the NHS now, because in the 2010 election campaign Cameron declared that there wouldn't be any, and neither he nor Lansley mentioned the 2007 document then either. But there it was. No one took it seriously enough.

In any case, the Health and Social Care Bill 2011 doesn't represent a major break with the policy of the Blair and Brown governments. The difference is that while New Labour ministers imagined a managed market, in which the government would tell investors the forms of health care they could provide, such as GP-led centres and APMS GP practices, Conservatives think investors should be left to decide for themselves what services to provide, and how. That was always going to happen, in one way or another, once the market principle was adopted. Nicholas Timmins summarized it accurately: 'The NHS will in effect be turned from what is still, broadly, a managed system of healthcare into something much more like a regulated industry of competing providers – and one over which the Secretary of State will no longer have day-to-day control.'[11]

With Cameron and Lansley the direction of past policy finally comes into the open. They feel no ambivalence about promoting privatization. When a health company executive described their plan as 'a waltz towards the private sector' they didn't protest that it wasn't.[12] When Lansley announced that the National Institute for Health and Clinical Excellence (NICE) would no longer have power to rule that a drug cannot be prescribed for NHS patients because its cost outweighs its benefits, he showed no embarrassment. He knew he would be seen as having succumbed to lobbying and was letting loose a massive increase in NHS spending, as drugs salespeople hastened to capitalise on the change. But his sympathies lay with the pharmaceutical industry. [13]

The decision to make the final push to privatization in the midst of savage public spending costs greatly increases the risk involved, even if the crisis can also be used as an excuse for ramming through the changes. Since late 2009 the number of job cuts throughout the NHS has mounted steadily, accompanied by the closure of wards and units, including A and E departments and maternity units; lengthening waiting lists and the return of bed blocking (as cuts to local authority budgets have reduced provision of the intermediate care needed by many patients on their discharge from hospital). Also re-emerging are shorter consultation times, notes lost, operations cancelled, more sick people left on corridor trolleys, sufferers from chronic illnesses marginalized, hospital infection rates rising again.[14]

In the short run Lansley's project is a reckless gamble with people's health. In the long run, it will give us something close to the most expensive and worst health system in the developed world, that of the USA: a low quality basic health service increasingly based, once more, on the ability to pay, with little or no accountability and exposed to serious risks of fraud and other harms. For the private sector it will be the bonanza that its spokesmen have openly campaigned for.

11

Defending the NHS

In January 2011, Eamonn Butler, the director of the Adam Smith Institute (and colleague of Dr Tim Evans, whom we first met negotiating the concordat with Alan Milburn), was asked whether he really thought that the NHS in England would now become a mere 'franchise'. His answer was revealing: 'It's been twenty years in the planning', he said. 'I think they'll do it' – simultaneously acknowledging the reality of the plot against the NHS, and dating its origins back to the early 1990s.[1]

But will 'they' be allowed to 'do it'? As the implications of the July 2010 White Paper sank in, almost every professional organization inside the NHS in England, or closely concerned with it, expressed strong criticisms that often seemed to verge on opposition. It was actively supported only by those with a financial stake in privatization – the commercial health lobby, and the 'entrepreneurial' GPs of the NHS Alliance. Organizations voicing serious concern included the Royal College of General Practitioners, the BMA, the Queen's Nursing Institute, the Patients' Association, the Commons Health Select Committee, the all-party parliamentary group for primary care and public health, the Community Practitioners and Health Visitors Association, the health service unions Unison and Unite, Cancer charities – even the Nuffield Trust. It would be hard to find a modern precedent for a major piece of legislation which was so universally condemned by everyone best qualified to understand it.[2]

But we should not overestimate the significance of all this. For some critics – the NHS Confederation, for example – the transformation of the NHS into a healthcare market is above all untimely: not something to undertake in the aftermath of a recession, or perhaps a continuing recession, but not necessarily a bad idea in itself. Others are mainly worried that the two projects – making cuts and reorganising the system – will be mutually damaging; they are not necessarily opposed to either the cuts or privatization in themselves.

But some of the Bill's most significant critics, including the Royal College of General Practitioners, who are at the centre of Lansley's plans, have focused primarily on the fact that the plans mean the end of the NHS as a public service. Dr Clare Gerada, who took over as president of the College in November 2010, thought that it meant 'the end of the NHS as we currently know it'. England's health system would, she believed, look more and more like America's – and GPs would be blamed for its failings.[3] But even though she spoke for a majority of GPs – fewer than a quarter of whom thought the plan would improve patient care –[4] she feared, and they feared, that if they carried their opposition too far the government might simply move directly to using private companies to commission care – in other words, to move even faster to full privatization. It was this consideration that led even GPs who were bitterly opposed to privatization to agree to join the new 'pathfinder' commissioning consortia that the government wanted set up in preparation for the implementation of the Health and Social Care Bill. They joined in order to try to keep control in their hands, rather than see it go directly into the hands of profit-oriented corporations.

As for opposition by the Labour leadership, it has been distinctly muffled. Blair's former health adviser Julian Le Grand (Simon Stevens' successor) declared, as a faithful Blairite, that Lansley's plans were simply 'a logical, sensible extension of those put in place by Tony Blair'.[5] In the second reading of the Health Bill, Labour's shadow Health Secretary, John Healey, put forward a cogent and detailed critique of the Bill but fell short of offering to do more than 'explain and expose the gap between what Ministers are saying and what they are doing in every debate at every stage of this legislation'.[6] He was handicapped by Labour's complicity in so much that had gone before.

In the end it will be up to the great majority of the public, who rely on the NHS, to stand up and fight for it. Ever since the marketization process began in earnest in 2000, and in some cases well before that, numerous organizations have been resisting it and trying to uphold the values and principles on which the NHS was founded. The list includes Keep Our NHS Public, Health Emergency, the NHS Support Federation, the NHS Consultants Association, and a host of groups and campaigns, sometimes supported by Unison or Unite, fighting to defend local NHS services.

Until Lansley's White Paper of July 2010, all these campaigns were met at the national level with a large degree of public apathy. But since 2010, and in the new era of mass mobilizations of public opinion, from the students in London to the protesters in Tunisia, Egypt and Libya, the mood has changed. Paul Corrigan, a former adviser to successive Labour health ministers, confidently assured readers of his blog: 'Governments with majorities don't publish Bills that don't become Acts. This Bill will become an Act.'[7] Maybe so, but by the time it reaches the end of its passage through both Houses of Parliament it could look different in key respects. And it remains to be seen how long Lansley's Liberal-Democrat allies will endure being seen as co-responsible for the results.

And how long will the measures in the Bill survive if it is passed? What may the Labour leadership find it necessary to promise, if opposition to the legislation among the public is sufficiently widespread, and profoundly felt? In his first comments on the issue since becoming leader, addressing the Welsh Labour Party Conference in February 2011, Ed Miliband denounced the Bill but stopped short of any commitment to repeal it.[8] A sufficiently strong and focused public reaction in England could stiffen Labour's resolve. The cuts that were beginning to be implemented seem bound to work in this direction.

The impact of the cuts

Wholesale reductions of hospital services in one major hospital after another were announced. In February 2011 St George's Hospital in south London announced that 500 jobs would go, including both nurses and consultants, and that three wards with 100 beds would close, including more than a quarter of the hospital's maternity beds. Kingston Hospital in south-west London announced the cutting of 20 per cent of its staff over the next five years. Southend University Hospital was to shed 400 jobs and close six wards. In the first seven weeks of 2011 over 3,000 NHS job losses were announced across London alone.[9] A TUC-funded study found that 53,000 NHS jobs were already scheduled to go throughout the UK.[10]

The impact was beginning to be felt in primary care too. Redbridge Primary Care Trust told GPs that they could only make four referrals a week. NHS South West Essex had sent

GPs a list of 213 procedures it would no longer normally fund. Other PCTs were using 'gateway' services to vet GP referrals and deny a significant number.[11] Just as Dr Gerada feared, it looked as if the new GP commissioning consortia were going to be rationing consortia.

Within the BMA a strong challenge emerged to the leadership's position of 'critical engagement' with the government's plans, and a demand for outright opposition. The development of serious opposition from a large part of the medical profession, and especially from GPs, was significant, because Lansley constantly claimed to have their support.

The false case for the Health and Social Care Bill

The government's claim that the NHS was in urgent need of further fundamental reform was also becoming more and more obviously false. During the previous ten years, while the NHS was being covertly marketized, the Labour government had raised NHS funding rapidly towards the average level of spending of the other major countries of western Europe. Spending on the NHS still remained significantly below that of the richer EU nations, and a significant portion of the new funding was absorbed by the costs of market creation. But the extra cash also produced some important improvements. Staff levels were improved, waiting times for elective care were sharply reduced, facilities were renovated or replaced.

This was reflected in the high marks given to the NHS in the Commonwealth Fund report cited in chapter 1. And by 2010 the particular charge constantly made by the marketizers, that England lagged behind European countries in the survival rates for major killer illnesses, was ceasing to be true.[12] Lansley repeatedly declared that a wholesale restructuring of the NHS was 'a necessity, not an option', and David Cameron asserted that 'pretending that there is some "easy option" of sticking with the status quo... is a complete fiction.'[13] But in January 2011, coinciding with the publication of the Health and Social Care Bill, a paper by the King's Fund economist John Appleby, published in the *BMJ*, showed that the marketizers' charge was unfounded. It turned out to rest partly on the use of European data that were not comparable with the English data (and in some cases highly unreliable), and partly on selecting static data instead of trends over time. For several of the conditions usually cited English survival rates have in fact been improving so fast over the last 30 years that if the trends continue they will overtake European rates by 2012.[14]

The real choice

The choice is not between change and no change. It is between handing over a public service to be developed by private enterprise in the 'interests of shareholders, and ensuring that it develops in the interests of the public – and as the public sees those interests, not as politicians declare them to be. To maintain that there is no capacity for improvement within public provision is empty rhetoric. What evidence is there that public services are incapable of change and improvement (provided they are not undermined by financial starvation or market-driven disorganization)?

Around the world there are various examples of excellent public and publicly-provided health services, and all of them need to be studied for ideas about ways to improve the NHS in England – and beginning with an examination of those that are developing within the UK itself. The national media largely ignore what occurs across our nearest borders, but what is happening there, and especially in Scotland and Wales, raises crucially important questions about the future now being charted for the NHS in England.[15]

Looking at Scotland

Even before devolution health ministers in Westminster had been too aware of Scottish sentiment to risk pushing the internal market very far there, and the Labour-Liberal Democrat coalition governments that held office in Scotland after devolution, from 1999 to 2007, recognised that voters would not support them if they followed England's path to a healthcare market. Scotland's Area Health Boards remained in place, foundation trust status was not introduced, nor was payment by results. The PFI was used for three Scottish hospital-building schemes, and one Independent Sector Treatment Centre was opened at Stracathro in Angus. But these measures provoked intense controversy and in 2003, responding to pressure from both doctors and the public, the coalition government ended the purchaser-provider split, restoring direct administration of the NHS in Scotland and decisively closing off the market option. Also in response to public opinion, in 2002 the Scottish Labour-Lib Dem coalition made personal care for the elderly free, instead of means-tested as in England.

The 2007 elections, however, led to the formation of a minority SNP government, and yet further departures from the market-driven policy that was being pursued in England. In 2008 hospital car parking charges – a significant deterrent for families – were abolished, except at PFI hospitals, where legal reasons prevented it; and in 2010 plans were announced to abolish prescription charges from 2011. No further PFI schemes have been undertaken. Glasgow's biggest acute hospital is being built with public funds, the ISTC at Stracathro was taken into public ownership, and plans to outsource the management of a health centre in Lanarkshire to a private company were dropped. Out-of-hours care is publicly provided.

Perhaps most significant of all for the future, in 2009 elections were introduced for the majority of the members of Scotland's Health Boards, beginning with two pilot schemes, to be evaluated after four years. This means that in addition to professional medical judgement democratic representation, rather than individual 'patient choice', could become a significant element in determining the direction of future change.

In face of all this the marketizers inevitably portray Scotland's NHS as a failure, with the usual misuse of statistics to support their claim. For example they routinely state that Scotland's waiting times are worse than England's, because no element of competition has been introduced in Scotland. In fact an analysis of newly-consolidated data concludes that since 2005 waiting times have fallen faster in Scotland than in England. In each year since then Scotland has actually had either the second shortest or (more often) the shortest waiting times of the four nations of the UK.[16] And over the ten years from 1999 to 2008 Scotland's mortality rates for all causes of death declined almost exactly as fast as England's.[17] As Dr Matthew Dunnigan, the author of the waiting times analysis, says, the objective comparison of English health statistics with those for the three devolved nations is now a very important task.

Looking at Wales

The story in Wales has many similarities to Scotland's. For the first eight years following devolution a Labour minority government was in office, only giving way to a Labour-Plaid Cymru coalition in 2007. But as in Scotland, even the initial Labour-led Welsh Assembly Government did not dare follow the English path. The purchaser-provider split remained, but Wales did not adopt foundation trusts or payment by results. Development remained based on collaboration and planning, rather than on a market system with legally enforceable contracts and all the tensions and extra administrative costs involved.

And after 2007, under the Labour-Plaid coalition, the purchaser-provider split itself was dropped. In 2009 a major reform resulted in the formation of just seven integrated Local Health Boards to plan and operate the NHS in Wales. These are very like the Area Health Boards in Scotland, but also have overall responsibility for all aspects of health, including public health, with a strong emphasis on linking health and social care.

The Local Health Boards in Wales are not elected but they must have members representing local primary care, community care, public health, local government and voluntary organizations, as well as lay members. In one Local Health Board (Powys) the purchaser-provider split was abolished earlier and the Board was integrated with primary care and community health service providers. Other Boards are set to follow suit – exactly the opposite direction of change from that taken in England, where even community health services have been forced into the marketplace.

Wales also declined to use the PFI for hospital-building, led

152

the way (in 2007) in abolishing prescription charges, abolished hospital parking charges, and dealt with the vexed issue of means-tested personal care for the elderly by widening the definition of what is considered nursing care (and therefore free), and by setting a flat-rate contribution to the cost of personal care throughout the whole country.

Considerations for England

We need to ask ourselves why Scotland and Wales opted to keep the NHS as a public service, and even extended the principle of free access. Longstanding Scottish and Welsh cultural traditions are certainly important, especially a deeply-embedded commitment to social democracy in public life, and in the medical profession, which politicians of all parties have to respect. But another key reason is cost. Next to education health is by far the most important and expensive devolved public service. Even before the financial crisis politicians of all parties in Scotland and Wales realised that if they followed the English route, and allowed the costs of operating a market to start soaking up ten per cent or more of the health budget, health services would be liable to deteriorate, with dire political consequences for themselves.

They know that the public spending cuts imposed by the government in Westminster will hit Scottish and Welsh health services. But they also know that the effects will be smaller than they would have been had they opted for a market, and that whatever they have to do will have a legitimate foundation in public opinion, which remains at the base of decision-making about the NHS in both countries. And when the crisis has passed they will still have a public health service, not a three-tiered healthcare market and a low-risk playground for healthcare corporations and 'doctorpreneurs'.

Scotland and Wales don't exhaust the alternatives for the future in England. Other good models of publicly-provided health services exist and deserve study. But the successful evolution of the NHS in the rest of the UK shows that Cameron's assertion that 'we can't afford not to modernise' – meaning that we have no alternative but to accept the abolition of the NHS as a public service – is pure bluster. It has no foundation in evidence and serves no interest except that of the private health industry. In the parts of the UK that the plot against the NHS couldn't reach, people see through it. They know that good health care for all means excluding profit-making, and have shown that with sufficient public backing that principle can prevail. We need to insist that in England too the NHS is not for selling.

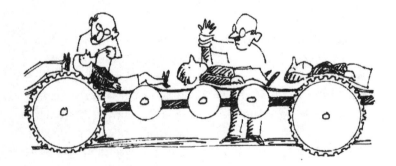

Notes

CHAPTER ONE

1 Interview with Colin Leys, 30 July 2000.

2 The implications of the Coalition's Health and Social Care Bill 2011 are spelled out in chapter 9.

3 Opinion polls can of course produce results tending to support a given view if the questions are designed to do so. The best evidence that people would reject an American style healthcare market is really the fact that the government have never asked for their opinion on it. But the basic finding of numerous polls is that most people want the NHS they have and are opposed to both competition and privatization.

4 *The NHS Plan: a plan for investment, a plan for reform*, CM 4818–I, 2000.

5 *The NHS Improvement Plan: Putting People at the Heart of Public Services*, CM 6268, 2004, p. 10. How other elements of the marketization agenda were handled in successive documents following up the NHS Plan is discussed in chapter 8.

6 http://news.bbc.co.uk/1/hi/health/4229791.stm

7 'Hewitt rules out limiting size of private sector role in NHS', *Guardian*, 20 September 2006.

8 Jenny Percival, 'NHS faces £65 bn bill for PFI hospitals', *Guardian*, 13 August 2010.

9 Jeremy Colman, quoted in the *Financial Times*, 5 June 2002.

10 See Allyson Pollock, *NHS plc*, Verso (second edition 2005), pages 13-14 and 249.

11 Hansard, HC Deb, 31 January 2011, c618).

12 HM Treasury, *Public Services: meeting the productivity challenge, a discussion document*, April 2003, especially pages 12-14. The document did not apply solely to health care.

13 Cathy Schoen, M.S., Robin Osborn, David Squires, Michelle M. Doty, Roz Pierson, and Sandra Applebaum, 'How Health Insurance Design Affects Access to Care and Costs, by Income, in Eleven Countries' *Health Affairs* Web First, November 18, 2010. A government spokesperson could only comment sourly that 'the UK lags behind many international healthcare

systems on survival rates – for example, for diseases such as cancer or stroke – and the NHS must reform in order to achieve better outcomes' (*Guardian* 19 November 2010) – as if that was quite sufficient to justify the government's latest privatization plans. It was later shown that the statistical basis for the government's statement was fallacious – a point taken up briefly in chapter 11.

CHAPTER TWO

1   The Cobden Centre is a charity funded and chaired by Toby Baxendale, a former food distributor, who describes himself as 'dedicated to furthering the teaching of the Austrian School of Economics and the revival of the Great Manchester School of Cobden and Bright'.

2   International comparisons have repeatedly found them to be among the highest, and sometimes the highest, in the world. See *Laing's Healthcare Market Review 2009-10*, Laing and Buisson 2009, pages 123-24.

3   *Financial Times*, 15 November 2007.

4   See Stewart Player and Colin Leys, *Confuse and Conceal: The NHS and Independent Treatment Centres*, Merlin Press, 2008, pages 48-51, and the oral evidence given to the Commons Health Committee by several clinicians, especially Mr Ian Leslie, president of the British Orthopaedic Association, the profession most concerned (Commons Health Committee, *Fourth Report of Session 2005-06*, Vol III, page 16).

5   A surcharge is a charge that may be levied to recover money that is reckoned to have been lost by a public servant through a dereliction of duty or abuse of office. In this instance the threat may have been idle, but felt real.

6   Survey of over 100 NHS chief executives by the *Health Service Journal*, cited in evidence to the Health Committee, Vol III, page 166.

7   According to a King's Fund briefing paper, by 2008 ISTCs had produced 85 per cent of the treatments they had been paid for, although only 25 per cent of the diagnostics. The paper did not say how much of the work had been done by NHS staff (Chris Naylor and Sue Gregory, *Independent Sector Treatment Centres*, the King's Fund, 2009, page 7).

8   For evidence on this see John Curtice and Oliver Heath, 'Do people want choice and diversity of proivision in public services?', in Alison Park, John Curtice, Katarina Thompson, Miranda Phillips and Ellizabeth Clery (eds), *British Social Attitudes: the 25th Report*, National Centre for Social

Research, 2009, pages 55-78. A YouGov poll for the BMA in June 2005 found that patients put clean hospitals and improved A and E at the top of their list of preferences, and choice bottom.

9   GPs in Tameside and Glossop were offered £130 for each such referral, and those in Ashton, Wigan and Leigh, £30. See Player and Leys, *Confuse and Conceal*, page 48.

10 David Amess, Conservative MP for Southend West, was the only MP whose patience gave out, telling his colleagues they were wasting their time.

11 Quality problems in ISTCs did improve when the bulk of their work came to be done by NHS surgeons.

12 *Financial Times*, 1 May 2007.

13 The current value of the shares in question had been far higher than this, and the gain to the backdaters and the loss to shareholders correspondingly much greater, at the time when they were backdated. The story is well documented on Wikipedia.

14 Jerome Mansmann, the CEO of Nation's Healthcare, which won three of the first ISTC contracts, explained to an Irish audience that there was a plan to create a market for private sector providers but that it looked 'unstated' ('Private healthcare opportunities for Ireland: an outsider's perspective', Nation's Healthcare slide presentation, nd).

15 John Carvel and Giles Tremlett, 'Milburn seeks role model in Spain', *Guardian*, 6 November 2001.

16 Manuel Martin-García and Marciano Sánchez Bayle, 'New forms of management and their impact on health inequalities', *Gaceta Sanitaria* 2004:18(Supl 1):96-1O1.

17 House of Commons *Debates*, 7 May 2003, col. 714.

18 Department of Health, *NHS Foundation Trusts*, *http://webarchive.nationalarchives.gov.uk/+/www.dh.gov.uk/en/Healthcare /Secondarycare/NHSfoundationtrust/index.htm*, accessed 3 January 2011. Labour ministers even claimed that they were a reincarnation of the traditions of the cooperative and mutualist movement.

19 See John Lister, *The NHS After 60*, Middlesex University Press, 2008, pages 158-9.

20 The total number of trusts has been diminishing through mergers. According to the NHS Confederation, which regularly updates its figures, early in 2011 there were 168 acute trusts of which 88 were foundation

trusts; 73 mental health trusts of which 37 were foundation trusts; plus 12 ambulance trusts and ten care trusts. See
http://www.nhsconfed.org/OurWork/political-engagement/Pages/NHS-statistics.aspx

CHAPTER THREE

1   See Allyson Pollock, *NHS plc: The Privatization of our Health Care*, Verso, second edition, 2005, page 40.

2   *The NHS Plan* paragraphs 8.19 and 8.24

3   The National Audit Office and the Commons Public Accounts committee reported in April and October 2007 respectively, and reached very similar conclusions.

4   Penny Dash, 'Plan B on the consultant contract', *Guardian*, 1 November 2002.

5   Donna Wright, 'People: Penny Dash MBA '94', *Stanford Business* May 2001, 69/3

6   Alan Milburn, presenting the second reading of the Health and Social Care Bill in the House of Commons, *Hansard*, 7 May 2003, col. 709.

7   'FTN statement on change to employment within the NHS', *Guardian* 28 January 2010.

8   House of Commons Committee of Public Accounts, *NHS Pay Modernization: New contracts for General Practice services in England*, Forty–first Report of Session 2007–08, 23 June 2008.

9   Interview with the BBC News website, January 19 2007, at http://news.bbc.co.uk/1/hi/health/6276793.stm

10   National Audit Office, *The Provision of Out-of-Hours Care in England*, HC 1041 2005-2006, 5 May 2006.

11   Take Care Now, a private limited company apparently belonging to Harmoni, the largest private provider of out of hours services, subsequently reappeared as Suffolk Integrated Healthcare.

12   In 2010 Sainsbury's looked like being the first brand name to make a success of this model, simply offering GPs free accommodation and some office services in Sainsbury's stores and expecting to make a profit from the extra business patients would bring in when visiting the surgery ('Sainsbury's offers GPs free premises as it launches national network of practices', *Pulse*, 26 November 2010).

13   'Private firms overtake GP consortiums in Darzi bids', *Pulse*, 28 April 2010.

14 NHS Support Federation, *NHS Unlimited? Who runs our GP services*, Brighton, 2010.

15 See Virgin Assura website at http://www.assuramedical.co.uk/virgin-group-enters-healthcare-sector-with-majority-shareholding-in-assura-medical.aspx

16 *NHS Unlimited?*, page 1.

17 Hewitt tried to save face by saying that the deadline of December 2008 remained, while the Health Minister, John Hutton, told the Commons Health Committee that it didn't (see *Changes to Primary Care Trusts: Second Report of Session 2005-06*, pages 18-19).

18 PCTs were required to stop employing them by April 2011. Data collected by UNISON showed that by February 2011 ten per cent of community health staff had formed or joined social enterprises, seventy-seven per cent had joined or set up NHS trusts or foundation trusts, eight per cent had joined local authorities and three per cent had gone freelance.

CHAPTER FOUR

1 *Sunday Times*, 7 March 2010.

2 *Guardian*, 29 Dec 2007.

3 *A Framework for Action*, Healthcare for London, 2007, pages 10-11.

4 *NHS Plan*, page 18.

5 Steve Nowottny, 'Revealed: NHS secretly wooed private firms over polyclinics', *Pulse*, 17 October 2009.

6 *Our NHS, Our Future, Next Stage Review Interim Report*, Department of Health, 2007, page 6.

7 *Our NHS, Our Future*, page 30.

8 The breakdown was Independent Sector, 31; 'consortia', 25; 3rd Sector/Social Enterprise, 21; GPs, 45; Others, including PCT provider arms, 8; Department of Health, FOI Reference Number DE585606, 28 January 2011

9 'Virgin Healthcare was advised to target "lucrative" young patients', *Pulse*, 24 June 2008.

10 Sue Hessel, 'Haringey's lost hospitals + health facts', presentation to the Radical History Network, Tottenham, 9 September 2009, drawing on Haringey PCT Annual Accounts 2008/09. Hessel estimated that the total annual cost to the PCT of leasing the premises was closer to £1.5 million.

11 Mike Broad, 'Government signals an end to Darzi centres', *Hospital*

Doctor, 4 February 2011, and letter from Dame Barbara Hakin to all PCTs in England, 3 February 2011.

12 See *Laing's Healthcare Market Review 2009-10*, page 225.

13 PCTs were paying GP led centres £180 per patient in the first year, compared with an average of £63 per patient for regular general practices (*Pulse*, 3 July 2009).

14 Ian Quin, 'Government dumps Darzi centres', *Pulse*, 3 February 2011.

15 The background to Hinchingbrooke's debt is given in Lister, *The NHS After 60*, page 194.

16 'Hingchingbrooke deal "just the start", says Britnell, *HealthInvestor*, February 2010.

17 Sally Gainsbury, 'NHS failure regime: up to 92 trusts may be culled', *Health Service Journal*, 18 September 2008.

18 Owen Bowcott, 'NHS advised to lose one in 10 workers', *Guardian*, 2 September 2009. The claim that Britnell had no authority to commission it looks like ministerial spin: see for example *OperatingTheatre Journal*, 7 September 2009:'Attempting to distance themselves from the report, ministerial sources suggested the review had been commissioned without full ministerial authority'.

19 According to the *Evening Standard* (9 September 2009) KPMG had 'significantly trumped' Britnell's Department of Health salary of £235,000 a year. As for his garden leave, it is 'the term given to a situation whereby an employee is required to serve out a period of notice at home (or "in the garden"). During this period the employee continues to receive all salary and benefits but is prohibited from commencing employment with new employers until the gardening leave period has expired' ('UK Employment Law' by Laytons Solicitors, at http://www.roydens.co.uk/content11.htm)

20 *NHS Chief Executive's Annual Report 2008-2009*, 20 May 2009, p. 47.

21 Sally Gainsbury, 'SHAs plan staff cuts of up to 10 pc', *Health Service Journal*, 4 February 2010.

22 Fiona Barr, 'Nicholson tells NHS doubters to go', *EHealth Insider*, 23 November 2010, at http://www.ehi.co.uk/news/primary-care/6447

CHAPTER FIVE

1   Richard G A Feachem, Neelam K Sekhri, Karen L White, Jennifer Dixon, Donald M Berwick, and Alain C Enthoven, 'Getting more for their dollar: a comparison of the NHS with California's Kaiser Permanente', *BMJ*, 19

January 2002. Dixon was then director of policy at the King's Fund and later became director of the Nuffield Trust.

2   Over seventy rapid responses were received by the journal pointing out the flawed nature of the analysis. See also Alison Talbot-Smith, Shamini Gnani, Allyson M Pollock andDenis Pereira Gray, 'Questioning the claims from Kaiser', *British Journal of General Practice*, 1 June 2004.

3   'Kaiser Permanente', *Healthcare Market News*, August 2002.

4   House of Commons Health Committee, *Second Report*, 1 February 2007.

5   Birmingham East and North NHS Primary Care Trust, 'Strategic Plan 2008-2011', September 2008.

6   Stephen Shortt and Dr Stephen Fowlie, 'Removing the policy barriers to integrated care', Nuffield Trust, 26 November 2009.

7   The National Leadership Network consisted of 150 health policy makers, management consultants, NHS Trust and private healthcare executives, as well as clinicians, professional leaders and regulators, mandated to 'provide collective leadership for the next phase of transformation, advise Ministers on developing policies and promote shared values and behaviours'. See note 10.

8   Oliver Wright, 'Doctors seek early retirement to avoid NHS work pressures', *Times*, 7 August 2003.

9   'Stressed consultants eye NHS exit', *Healthcare Market News*, August 2003.

10 NHS National Leadership Network Local Hospitals Project, 'Strengthening Local Services: The Future of the Acute Hospital – Reference and Resource Report', 21 March 2006.

11 Jo Ellins and Chris Ham, 'NHS Mutual: Engaging staff and aligning incentives to achieve higher levels of performance', Nuffield Trust, July 2009.

12 Department of Health, 'Integrated care pilots expansion', Gateway reference 13542, 4 February 2010.

13 House of Commons Health Committee, *NHS Next Stage Review: First Report of Session 2008-09*, 15 December 2009.
    http://www.publications.parliament.uk/pa/cm200809/cmselect/cmhealth/5 3/5308.htm,

14 Five of the 16 integrated care pilot sites were in the same areas as provisional pilots for personal health budgets. By November 2010, 31 sites have been awarded full pilot status and the new Health and Social Care Bill fully supports the extension of personal budgets. Indeed 18 of the

above sites are now also piloting direct payments for health care, a move that was also anticipated by the previous government. see Nicola Watt, Department of Health,' Personal health budgets: helping to build a more responsive, more integrated, NHS',

http://www.wsdactionnetwork.org.uk/news/features/personal_health.html

15 Italics added: see Birmingham East and North NHS Primary Care Trust, 'Birmingham East and North and Solihull, Local Health Economy Overarching Vision and Plans 2008-2013'.

16 'Insurance firms eye top-up opportunities', *Healthcare Market News*, December 2008.

17 'PCTs must provide clarity on top-ups', *Healthcare Market News*, March 2009.

18 'BUPA Insurance adopts controversial clinical guidelines', *Healthcare Market News*, November 2006.

19 'Consultants remain opposed to care management proposals', *Healthcare Market News*, March 2009.

20 The 14 were: Aetna; AXA PPP; BUPA; CHKS; Dr Foster; Health Dialog Services Corporation; Humana; KPMG LLP; McKesson; McKinsey; Navigant Consulting; Tribal; UnitedHealth Europe; and WG Consulting.

21 *Healthcare Market News*, March 2009.

22 Ian Quinn,'Pioneering pathfinder consortium signs referral management deal with UnitedHealth UK, *Pulse*, 8 December 2010.

CHAPTER SIX

1 Tash Shifrin, 'PFI to cost £40bn over next five years', *Public Finance*, 11 February 2010.

2 'What lies beneath?' *HealthInvestor*, 8 September 2010.

3 Laing & Buisson, Laing's Healthcare Market Review 2009-2010', page 105.

4 'A little more conversation: GHG's "manifesto" raises valid points, but also reveals the firm's public sector ambitions', *HealthInvestor*, 6 May 2010.

5 The source for this and the following paragraph is David Smith, 'South African hospital firm admits "cash for kidney" transplants', *Guardian*, 10 November 2010.

6 *Laing's Healthcare Market Review 2009-2010*, page 105.

7 See note 6.

8 Owen Bowcott, 'Hospital closures inevitable over next five years', *Guardian*, 14 January 2010.

9   'Running circles', *HealthInvestor*, 13 April 2010.

10   Sarah Utecht, 'In practice', *HealthInvestor*, 8 August 2010.

11   John Elledge, 'Virgin reveals its primary care plan', *GPonline*, 18 January 2008.

12   Ian Quinn, 'Virgin Healthcare says 300 practices tempted to join network', *Pulse*, 19 May 2008.

13   'The second coming', *HealthInvestor*, 5 March 2010

14   *HealthInvestor* thought the primary care sector would have to follow the example of dentistry. Dentists may 'form "Dental Body Corporates", which allows firms to carry out the business of dentistry under certain stipulations'. ('The Second Coming').

15   The partnerships, known as 'GPCos', had either won, or secured preferred bidder stage for, 68 health centres which were expected to deliver annual revenues of £60m.

16   David Craig, *Plundering the Public Sector: How New Labour are letting consultants run off with £70 billion of our money*, Constable, 2006, page 41.

17   'Penny Dash, Partner McKinsey: HealthInvestor Power Fifty 2010', *HealthInvestor*, November 2010.

18   'The rail billionaires', *The Economist*, 1 July 1999, http://www.economist.com/node/218876/comments; and Clayton Hirst, 'The might of the McKinsey mob', *Independent on Sunday* 20 January 2002.)
     http://www.independent.co.uk/news/business/analysis-and-features/the-might-of-the-mckinsey-mob-664081.html

19   John Lister, 'London's NHS on the Brink', *BMA*, 6 January 2010.

20   Helen Mooney, 'McKinsey accused of unfair advantage on commissioning', *Health Service Journal*, 5 October 2006.

21   Helen Mooney, 'McKinsey "PCT support" bid sparks conflict of interest row', *Health Service Journal*, 21 September 2006.

22   Andy Cowper, 'World class commissioning: quality assurance', *Health Service Journal*, 9 June 2008.

23   In a mixture of basic salary, various awards, and through exercising stock options: see David Phelps, 'Minnesota's highest-paid CEO: $102 million' *Minneapolis Star Tribune*, 30 June 2010.

24   Peter Latman, 'UnitedHealth CEO McGuire Gives Back $620 Million', WSJ Law Blog, *Wall Street Journal*, 7 December 2007. The affair is well covered in Wikipedia as well as on numerous websites.

25 Hugh Gravelle, Mark Dusheiko, Rod Sheaff, Penny Sargent, Ruth Boaden, Susan Pickard, Stuart Parker, Martin Roland. 'Impact of case management (Evercare) on frail elderly patients: controlled before and after analysis of quantitative outcome data', *BMJ*, 15 November 2006.

26 UnitedHealth, 'NHS South Central Specialised Commissioning Group', April 2009.
http://www.unitedhealthuk.co.uk/OurWork/SouthCentralSCG.aspx

27 'National Association of Primary Care (NAPC) and United Health UK launch first how-to guide for GP consortia', National Association of Primary Care, October 10 2010.

28 Steffie Woolhandler and David U. Himmelstein, 'Competition in a publicly funded healthcare system', *BMJ*, 29 November 2007.

CHAPTER SEVEN

1 House of Commons Health Committee, *The Use of Management Consultants by the NHS and the Department of Health*, 5th Report of Session 2008-09. In 2007-08 the total was over £300m, not counting spending by foundation trusts. In 2008-09 the Department of Health alone spent £204 million on consultancy from some 90 companies, while its IT project, Connecting for Health, spent a further £38 million. (http://www.dh.gov.uk/en/FreedomOfInformation/Freedomofinformation publicationschemefeedback/FOIreleases/DH_103938.)

2 David Craig, *Plundering the Public Sector: How New Labour are letting consultants run off with £70 billion of our money*, Constable 2006, page 229.

3 Not counting the substantial costs involved in learning to use it if it ever does work. The Wikipedia entry on Connecting for Health is unusually specific and details the companies that have been sacked or have withdrawn along the way, the secrecy surrounding the programme and the mass of expert criticism to which it has been subjected. It appears a classic example of why an estimated 73 per cent of large IT projects fail (see the entertaining diagnosis of the reasons for this in Craig's book *Plundering*, chapter 10).

4 *Partnerships for Prosperity: the Private Finance Initiative*, Treasury Taskforce, 1997, page 1, cited in Sally Ruane, 'Corporate and political strategy in relation to the Private Finance Initiative in the UK', *Critical Social Policy*, 105, 2010, Vol 30(4).

5   Summarized in Paul Gosling, 'The rise of the "public services industry"', a report for UNISON, September 2009, p. 29.

6   Jon Ungoed-Thomas, Claire Newell and Holly Watt, 'Ex-ministers cash in on days of power', *Sunday Times*, 24 February 2008. At that time 18 New Labour ex-ministers had taken private sector jobs.

7   Paul Gosling, 'The rise of the "public services industry"', a report for UNISON, September 2009, and Craig, *Plundering*, pages 164-68.

8   http://www.tribalgroup.co.uk/?id=66&ob=2&rid=223S.

9   For this and several similar cases see David Rowland, 'The interface between the Department of Health and private companies with contracts to provide services on behalf of the NHS', unpublished paper, n.d. See also Paul Gosling, 'The rise of the "public services industry"'.

10   Data from the website of DHF and from Rowland, 'The interface'.

11   The information in this section is mainly drawn from the Charity Commission's website.

12   Scott L.Greer and Holly Harman, *The Department of Health and the Civil Service*, The Nuffield Trust, January 2007.

13   Only the Social Market Foundation had a mix of funding similar to that of the King's Fund, though on a much smaller scale and with only a partial interest in health policy: in 2009 £783,000 out of total revenues of £914,000 came from 'charitable activities', i.e. 'conference and event sponsorship' and 'research projects sponsorship'.

14   'NHS Alliance's response to the White Paper', press release 12 July 2010; and 'GP commissioning takes hold', press release, 17 January 2011. An even more whole-hog supporter of GP commissioning is the National Association for Primary Care, a GP-led and pharmaceutical-supported pressure group.

15   Denis Campbell, 'NHS White Paper proposals backed by only one in four doctors', *Guardian*, 24 October 2010.

16   Fundholding anticipated GP commissioning consortia. GPs could apply to administer a fixed annual budget for the average needs of their registered patients for secondary care. Before the incoming Labour government abolished it, 60 per cent of GPs had become fundholders.

17   See http://www.powerbase.info/index.php/Health_Portal, and especially the film by Tamasin Cave and David Miller: 'The Health Industry Lobbying Tour'.

18   See Centre for Health Leadership and Enterprise at the University of

Cambridge Judge Business School, Outreach: Cambridge Health Network, http://www.health.jbs.cam.ac.uk/corporate/outreach.html. What the American conglomerate Halliburton is doing in this company would be interesting to know.

19 Tamasin Cave, 'Nurses for Reform', *BMJ* 2010; 340:c1371.

20 http://www.nursesforreformblog.com/2008/06/19/nurses-group-welcomes-review-to-usher-in-private-top-ups-2/

21 http://www.spinwatch.org.uk/blogs-mainmenu-29/tamasin-cave-mainmenu-107/5391-private-health-lobby-out-in-force-at-tory-conference

CHAPTER EIGHT

1   Scott L.Greer and Holly Jarman, *The Department of Health and the Civil Service: From Whitehall to Department of Delivery to Where?*, The Nuffield Trust, 2007.

2   *The NHS Improvement Plan*, pages 11 and 53.

3   See George Monbiot, 'Labour's perverse polyclinic scheme is the next step in privatising the NHS', *Guardian*, 29 April 2008).

4   That is, they would be Alternative Provider Medical Services contracts. These could be given to non-profit social enterprises, but in practice they were expected to go to either corporate providers or groups of 'entrepreneurial' GPs.

5   The aim had been revealed a year before in an internal circular issued by the Chief Executive of the NHS, Sir Nigel Crisp. The reaction to it within the NHS at the time was one of the reasons for his departure in March 2006: see John Lister, *The NHS After 60*, Middlesex University Press, 2008, pages 171-77.

6   Susan Mayor, 'GPs challenge London PCTs as practice contracts go to private companies', *BMJ* 336:412, 21 February 2008. UnitedHealth was also awarded a GP contract in Derby itself.

7   http://www.healthdirect.co.uk/tag/pfi .

8   *High Quality Care for All*, pages 16-17.

9   *Creating a patient led NHS* para 3.6.

10 Andrew Corbett-Nolan, 'Enterprise Value', *HealthInvestor* 5 February 2009.

11 John Curtice and Oliver Heath, 'Do people want choice and diversity of provision in public services?', in Alison Park, John Curtice, Katarina Thompson, Miranda Phillips and Elizabeth Clery (eds), *British Social Attitudes: the 25th Report* 2009, pages 55-78. It is relevant that another 2009

study, not cited by the White Paper, found little evidence to support the White Paper's contention that providers respond competitively to the choices exercised by patients and their GPs (Anna Dixon and others, *How Patients Choose and How Providers Respond*, King's Fund, 2009).

12 'Doctors claim study on patient choice suppressed', *Guardian* 1 January 2007. Another survey for the Healthcare Commission found that choice of hospital and even choice of admission date were of so little interest to patients that it was not worth including questions about choice in the Commission's next survey of hospitals' performance ('Hospital choice irrelevant, say patients', *Guardian*, 14 March 2007).

13 Department of Health, Social Enterprise in the NHS, http://www.dh.gov.uk/en/Managingyourorganization/Socialenterprise/NHS/index.htm

14 http://www.socialenterprise.org.uk/data/files/stateofsocialenterprise2009.pdf The survey was conducted by a private firm, CELLO mruk research. After identifying the total of 5,355 social enterprises it conducted telephone interviews with 962 'senior figures' in these organizations and extrapolated the results to the total population of 5,355.

15 It looks as if it may have been arrived at as follows. The Coalition's report mentions in passing an estimate by the Department for Business of 62,000 social enterprises in the UK in 2007-08 (Williams, M. and Cowling, M., 2009, *Annual Small Business Survey 2007/08*, Department for Business, Enterprise and Regulatory Reform). Of the 5,355 social enterprises sampled in the Coalition's survey, nine per cent said they were concerned with 'health and social care'; and nine per cent of 62,000 is about 6,000.

16 Patient and public involvement in developing primary medical services Department of Health – Health care.mht

17 *Strengthening Accountability: Involving Patients and the Public*, Department of Health, 2003, http://www.dh.gov.uk/prod_consum_dh/groups/dh_digitalassets/@dh/@en/documents/digitalasset/dh_4074292.pdf

18 Ipsos Mori were asked to analyze the results and perhaps surprisingly agreed. See Jessica Elgood, Research Director Ipsos Mori, *Healthcare for London: Consulting the Capital, Analysis of responses, www.healthcareforlondon.nhs.uk/assets/...the.../Ipsos-Mori-presentation.ppt*

19 Joint Overview and Scrutiny Committee (JOSC) to review 'Healthcare for

London', Final Report of the Committee April 2008,
http://www.healthcareforlondon.nhs.uk/assets/Publications/Consulting-
the-Capital/JOSC-to-review-Healthcare-for-London.pdf

20 Healthcare for London, *Consulting the Capital*,
http://www.healthcareforlondon.nhs.uk/consulting-the-capital/#section3

21 'Patient power sees off giant', *Pulse*, 7 September 2006.

22 See Ursula Pearce's detailed review of the law on public consultation in
2008 at
http://www.keepournhspublic.com/pdf/UrsulaPearcePublicConsultationN
HSNov2008-2.pdf

23 The *Independent*'s Nina Lakhani has covered a series of these. According
to her article of 1 November 2009, NHS trusts have paid 'millions' of
pounds to settle court cases with suspended or dismissed doctors and
nurses and secure their silence: http://www.independent.co.uk/life-
style/health-and-families/health-news/nhs-is-paying-millions-to-gag-whist
leblowers-1812914.html

24 By 2009 even George Osborne as Conservative shadow chancellor said it
was 'totally discredited'(*Observer*, 15 November 2009).

25 The story is told in Allyson Pollock, *NHS Plc: The Privatization of Our
Health Care*, Verso, second edition, 2005, pages 219-23.

CHAPTER NINE

1 Explanatory notes to Part 3 chapter 1 of the Health and Social Care Bill.

2 Explanatory notes.

3 Anna Dixon, the director of policy at the King's Fund, 'Competition versus
integration: how to get the balance right', The King's Fund, 21 February
2011, reporting on a discussion held with Penny Dash's Cambridge Health
Network. http://www.kingsfund.org.uk/blog/competition_versus.html

4 Ian Quinn, 'GP referrals clampdown "in breach" of competition rules',
Pulse, 24 February 2011.

5 Annex B of Sir David Nicholson's letter to all NHS leaders, 17 February
2011.

6 House of Commons Public Bill Committee: Health and Social Care Bill,
11 February 2011, question 395.

7 Public Bill Committee: Health and Social Care Bill, question 95.

8 *Achieving World Class Productivity in the NHS 2009/10 – 2013/14:Detailing
the Size of the Opportunity*, Department of Health and McKinsey and

Company, March 2009.

9   Steve Davies, *Contract Cleaning and Infection Control*, a report for
    UNISON, 2009.

10 See the chapter by David Rowland on 'Long-term care for older people' in
    Allyson Pollock, *NHS plc*, Verso (second edition 2005), pages 192-93.

11 Sarah Calkin, 'Lack of nurses on 111 line sparks safety fears', *Nursing
    Times*, 14 December 2010. Fewer than 17 per cent of the staff in one centre
    tasked with dealing with calls from patients were qualified nurses. For the
    reduction of the skill mix to pay for the high cost of PFI see Allyson M.
    Pollock, Matthew G. Dunnigan, Declan Gaffney, David Price and Jean
    Shaoul, 'Planning the "new" NHS: downsizing for the 21st century', *BMJ*,
    1999, 319: 179. On GP-led health centres see Gareth Iacobucci, 'Pulse
    investigation: new health centres are GP led in name only', *Pulse* 4
    February 2009.

12 *Care and Compassion? Report of Health Service Ombudsman on ten
    investigations into NHS care of older people*, Parliamentary and Health
    Service Ombudsman, February 2011.

13 Explanatory note 538 to Clause 56 of the Health and Social Care Bill.

14 *Focused on Better Care, Annual Report of the Care Quality Commission
    for 2009/10*, p. 5. The comparison is with the 2005 staffing of three previous
    organisations that were merged into the CQC.

15 Matthew Hill, 'Failing care homes may "slip net"', BBC News 9 November
    2010, http://www.bbc.co.uk/news/health-11709811

16 House of Commons Public Bill Committee: Health and Social Care Bill,
    11 February 2011, Questions 301 to 328.

17 Karen Bloor, Emma Harvey and Alan Maynard, 'NHS Management and
    Administration Staffing and Expenditure in a National and International
    Context', report for the Department of Health, University of York, 2005.
    The Department sat on the report for five years.

18 The minimum recommended size of risk pool is said to be 500,000. The
    average population covered by the pathfinder consortia listed by the
    Department of Health in December 2010 was closer to 150,000; see 'GP
    pathfinder consortia by Strategic Health Authority region', Department
    of Health, 9 December 2010, at
    http://www.dh.gov.uk/en/Aboutus/Features/DH_122384

19 Variations on this phrase are commonly heard in discussions of US health
    care. This one comes from Peter Phillips and Bridget Thornton, 'Practices

in Health Care and Disability Insurance: Delay, Diminish, Deny, and Blame', Sociology 436 class, Sonoma State University, spring 2007, with David Abbott, Brandon Beccio, Daniela Bravo, Laura Buck, Chris Castro, Andrew Kent, Chris Morello, Brian Murphy, Debra Sedeno, Kimberly Soho, and Yuri Wittman; available on the Keep Our NHS Public website.

20 McKesson press release January 12 2005; Karen Gullo, 'Ex-McKesson chairman McCall gets 10-year prison term for securities fraud', *Industry-News.org*, March 6 2010.

21 Marc Songini, 'McKesson to settle drug lawsuit with $350M payment', *Mass High Tech: The Journal of New England Technology*, 23 April 2009.

22 Anthony Barnett and Solomon Hughes, 'UK's elderly care plan run by "cheats"', *Observer* 10 November 2002..

23 'UnitedHealth Group Settles for $350 Million', Reuters, 13 January 2009.

24 Deena Beasley, 'California seeks to fine UnitedHealth up to $9.9 billion', Reuters 8 September 2010, at http://www.reuters.com/article/2010/09/08/us-unitedhealth-california-idUSTRE6873WB20100908

25 Richard Winton and Cara Mia DiMassa, 'Kaiser accepts patient dumping settlement', *Los Angeles Times*, 16 May 2007.

26 'Since 1986, almost $17 billion dollars have been returned to the U.S. Treasury in this way, and whistleblower rewards have exceeded $2.5 billion': see 'Justice Department joins McKesson whistleblower lawsuit', *Newsinferno*, 7 October 2008.

27 The decision in the Bettercare case in Northern Ireland suggests that an action of this kind would be likely to succeed under the provisions of the Health and Social Care Bill. See Allyson Pollock and David Price, 'The BetterCare judgment—a challenge to health care European competition law may cover publicly funded, privately provided care', *BMJ*, 2003; 326 : 236 doi: 10.1136/bmj.326.7383.236 (Published 1 February 2003)

CHAPTER TEN

1 Ian Quinn, 'Pioneering pathfinder consortium signs referral management deal with UnitedHealth UK', *Pulse*, 8 December 2010.

2 The evidence is memorably recorded in clip from the hearings included in Michael Moore's film *Sicko*. The doctor had worked for Aetna, one of the companies employed in England under the FESC.

3 Ian Quinn, 'GP links to private firms could derail consortia', *Pulse*, 20 October 2010.

4   Randeep Ramesh, 'NHS reform could see surgeries on stock market;, *Guardian* 2 March 2011.

5   See Diagnosis website http://www.diagnosisltd.eu/pubs.html; and Emma Stanton and Oliver Warren, 'Leadership opportunities for trainees', *BMJ Careers* 1 January 2011.

6   Hans-Ulrich Deppe, 'The nature of health care: commodification versus solidarity', in Leo Panitch and Colin Leys (eds), *Morbid Symptoms: Health Under Capitalism, Socialist Register 2010*, pages 29-38.

7   Dr Natalie-Jane MacDonald, quoted in Gareth Iacobucci, 'GPs face new hospital admission targets', *Pulse* 11 December 2007.

8   Susie Sell, 'GPs more likely to refer to private sector due to budget pressures', *Healthcarerepublic* 2 November 2010, at http://www.gponline.com/News/article/1038354/GPs-likely-refer-private-sector-due-budget-pressures/

9   Chris Blackhurst, 'If we want decent healthcare, it's time for us all to cough up', *London Evening Standard*, 16 February 2011.

10 E.g. Unison General Secretary Dave Prentis, 'The case for the NHS', *Guardian*, 13 October 2010.

11 Nicholas Timmins, 'Healthcare on the brink of a cultural revolution', *Financial Times*, 17 January 2010.

12 'Private firms plan to cash in on NHS shake-up', *The Mirror*, 29 December 2010.

13 Polly Toynbee, 'Forget patients. Andrew Lansley is the servant of big pharma', *Guardian*, 2 November 2010.

14 'Cut backs in social care will cause "major problems", the NHS Confederation has warned ahead of the comprehensive spending review', *Health Service Journal*, 18 October 2010. On the impact of job cuts on services by the autumn of 2010 see the *Sunday Telegraph*, 10 October 2010, and the *Independent*, 18 October 2010.

CHAPTER ELEVEN

1   Radio 4, 19 January:
    http://news.bbc.co.uk/today/hi/today/newsid_9366000/9366535.stm

2   The consultation on Lansley's July 2010 White Paper, which began ten days after the White Paper was published, on 22 July, in the middle of the summer holidays, and ended on October 11, barely allowed time for the professional organizations most concerned to reply to it. The BMA later

observed that the government's response to the consultation had in any case ignored virtually all the points made to it.

3   *Guardian* 19 November 2010.

4   Steve Nowottny, 'Profession unconvinced by White Paper reforms, King's Fund survey finds', *Pulse*, 26 October 2010.

5   *Financial Times*, 29 October 2010.

6   House of Commons *Hansard Debates*, 31 January 2011, col. 627.

7   'The winding future path for the Health and Social Care Bill', blog at *Health Matters*, 27 January 2011,
    http://www.pauldcorrigan.com/Blog/category/reform-of-the-nhs/

8   Posted on the New Statesman website 19 February 2011, at
    http://www.newstatesman.com/blogs/the-staggers/2011/02/labour-party-government-wales

9   *Guardian* 18 February 2011, citing Royal College of Nursing data.

10 'NHS to lose 50,000 jobs, trade unions say', BBC News, 23 February 2011,
    http://www.bbc.co.uk/news/uk-england-london-12548153

11 Ian Quinn, 'Radical new gateways reject one in eight GP referrals', *Pulse*, 23 February 2011. The report was based on 360 GP responses to a survey by the magazine, and Freedom of Information responses by 32 primary care organizations.

12 Department of Health. Ministerial briefing on the Health and Social Care Bill. 2011, in *Modernising the NHS the Health and Social Care Bill*, The Liberal Democrats Latest News Detail.mht

13 Nicholas Timmins and Jim :Packard, 'Reform a necessity, says Lansley', *Financial Times*, 20 January 2011; and Transcript of the Prime Minister's speech on modern public service, 17 January 2011,
    http://www.number10.gov.uk/news/speeches-and-transcripts/2011/01/prime-ministers-speech-on-modern-public-service-58858

14 John Appleby, 'Does poor health justify NHS reform?', *BMJ* 2011; 2011; 342:d566.

15 Northern Ireland has also declined to follow the market route, though from other considerations and historical traditions (see for instance the insightful overview by Northern Ireland's former Chief Medical Officer, Dr Henrietta Campbell, in Scott Greer and David Rowland (eds), *Devolving Policy, Diverging Values? The values of the United Kingdom's national health services*, The Nuffield Trust, 2007, pages 33-68). Serious

studies of what is happening to the NHS in Northern Ireland, and in Scotland and Wales, are urgently needed.

16 M G Dunnigan, personal communication; data based on Office for National Statistics, *UK Health Statistics 2010*, Tables 6.6a-f,Edition No 4.

17 M G Dunnigan, personal communication; data based on Office for National Statistics, *Regional Trends* (2001 and 2009), pages 36 and 41.

Index

Colin Leys is an emeritus professor at Queen's University Canada and an honorary professor at Goldsmiths College London. His books include *The Rise and Fall of Development Theory*, *Market-Driven Politics,* and *Total Capitalism*. He has been studying and writing about the NHS since the late 1990s.

Stewart Player is a public policy analyst with extensive experience of studying the NHS. He is the co-author with Colin Leys of *Confuse and Conceal: The NHS and Independent Treatment Centres* and an occasional contributor to *Private Eye.*